THE GREAT PHYSICIAN'S

 for

HEARTBURN AND ACID REFLUX

JORDAN RUBIN

with Joseph Brasco, M.D.

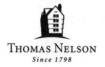

THOMAS NELSON
Since 1798

NASHVILLE   DALLAS   MEXICO CITY   RIO DE JANEIRO   BEIJING

Every effort has been made to make this book as accurate as possible. The purpose of this book is to educate. It is a review of scientific evidence that is presented for information purposes. No individual should use the information in this book for self-diagnosis, treatment, or justification in accepting or declining any medical therapy for any health problems or diseases. No individual is discouraged from seeking professional medical advice and treatment, and this book is not supplying medical advice.

Any application of the information herein is at the reader's own discretion and risk. Therefore, any individual with a specific health problem or who is taking medications must first seek advice from his personal physician or health-care provider before starting a health and wellness program. The author and Thomas Nelson Publishers, Inc., shall have neither liability nor responsibility to any person or entity with respect to loss, damage, or injury caused or alleged to be caused directly or indirectly by the information contained in this book. We assume no responsibility for errors, inaccuracies, omissions, or any inconsistency herein.

In view of the complex, individual nature of health problems, this book and the ideas, programs, procedures, and suggestions herein are not intended to replace the advice of trained medical professionals. All matters regarding one's health require medical supervision. A physician should be consulted prior to adopting any program or programs described in this book. The author and publisher disclaim any liability arising directly or indirectly from the use of this book.

Published in Nashville, Tennessee. Thomas Nelson is a trademark of Thomas Nelson, Inc.

Thomas Nelson Inc. titles may be purchased in bulk for educational, business, fundraising, or sales promotional use. For information, please e-mail SpecialMarkets@ThomasNelson.com.

Scripture quotations noted NKJV are from THE NEW KING JAMES VERSION. Copyright © 1982 by Thomas Nelson, Inc. Used by permission. All rights reserved.

Scripture quotations noted NIV are from the HOLY BIBLE: NEW INTERNATIONAL VERSION®. Copyright © 1973, 1978, 1984 by International Bible Society. Used by permission of Zondervan Publishing House. All rights reserved.

Scripture quotations noted KJV are from the KING JAMES BIBLE.

Library of Congress Cataloging-in-Publication Data

Rubin, Jordan.
    The Great Physician's Rx for heartburn and acid reflux / by Jordan Rubin with Joseph Brasco.
      p. cm.
    Includes bibliographical references
    ISBN-10: 0-7852-1934-X (hardcover)
    ISBN-13: 978-0-7852-1934-X (hardcover)
    1. Heartburn and Acid Reflux—Popular works. 2. Heartburn and Acid Reflux—Religious aspects—Christianity. 3. Heartburn and Acid Reflux—Rehabilitation—Popular works. I. Brasco, Joseph. II. Title.
RC660.4.R84 2006
616.4'6206—dc22   2005036830

Printed in the United States of America

07 08 09 10 QW 6 5 4 3 2 1

Contents

INTRODUCTION

A Bad Feeling After He Ate

Tim Roos is thirty-three years old, but during his twenties, this aspiring California farmer loved to attack the all-you-can-eat restaurants where he could really get his money's worth. One of his favorite places to gorge himself was a Chinese restaurant called the Four Seasons Buffet in his hometown of Modesto, California. Tim would graze the entire buffet line, returning several times to his table with plates piled high with the tangy and delicious entrées. "I would eat until I became uncomfortable," said Tim, a rugged, muscular type with calloused hands who stands six feet, four inches with 245 pounds filling out his frame.

After he and his buddies declared a truce with the buffet line, Tim's stomach would begin acting up. Within the hour, his bloated stomach felt like it had risen into his chest, which prompted incessant burping and expressions of "excuse me" to his friends. He suppressed gas as well.

The burning sensation in his chest, Tim figured, was heartburn. He also presumed that burping up his meal was symptomatic of acid reflux. The incidences of stomach distress increased throughout his twenties, but he never visited a doctor due to a streak of independence. You feel that way, he said, when you grow up as the son of a farmer in the San Joaquin Valley. To deal with his steady indigestion, he kept a stash of antacids in the house and in his truck.

Then Tim met Suzy Powell, a two-time Olympian who throws the discus for the United States. When they would go out on dates, Tim made sure they stayed away from his old buffet haunts, but he still experienced acid reflux after feasting on a steak dinner or an enchilada-and-burrito combination plate. "All I could do to put out the fire was throw a couple of Tums down the hatch," he said. "I tried to hide my acid reflux from Suzy. Believe me, it wasn't the most pleasant experience for her. I constantly burped when I took her home in my pickup truck. I must say that it didn't smell too good inside the closed cab."

Suzy must have not minded too much because she and Tim married two years ago. When they set up housekeeping together, they ate what they thought was a balanced diet. Nutrition has always been über-important to Suzy, a world-class athlete who's training to make the US Olympic team for the third time in 2008. Her engine demands plenty of protein, carbs, and vegetables.

Tim fell in right behind her, but even eating what most would consider a balanced diet failed to diminish the continuing episodes of heartburn and acid reflux. "I wasn't the type to run to the doctor," he said. "I grew up in a tough farming family, where we worked the land to grow almond trees. I spent my summers in the fields clearing brush, keeping the weeds down, trimming trees, and doing tractor work. I decided I was going to live with my heartburn and acid reflux because I didn't view it as a medical condition. I wasn't in an extreme amount of pain—just mild discomfort. I thought everyone experienced indigestion to one degree or another. Like the person who needs glasses, I figured everyone else couldn't see that well either."

Then in 2006, Tim and Suzy heard me share the message of the Great Physician's prescription at their church, Calvary Temple Worship Center, pastored by Glen Berteau. I had the privilege of ministering to the church body that Sunday morning, and the pastoral team and congregation responded so well that Calvary Temple hosted a "7 Weeks of Wellness" challenge to take the health of the congregation to the next level. More than 360 men and women participated, including Tim and Suzy.

Each week, they listened as Kelli Williams, the health ministries pastor and a registered nurse, utilized the 7 Weeks of Wellness church curriculum that's based on my foundational book, *The Great Physician's Rx for Health and Wellness.* Tim liked what he heard, and Suzy was on board as well since she was vitally interested in fine-tuning her body for international competition.

The couple had been eating fairly healthily before they heard me speak, and by most people's measuring sticks, they qualified for sainthood since they veered away from fast-food drive-thrus and shunned fried entrées at home and away. Yet they still ate rolls, bread, and pasta made from enriched white flour and supermarket meats produced from livestock or chickens that munched on adulterated feed pumped up with antibiotics or growth hormones.

Tim and Suzy decided to follow the Great Physician's prescription and eat foods that God created in a form healthy for the body. They shopped for organic alternatives and filled their refrigerator and cupboard with grass-fed beef, free-range poultry, bread and pasta produced from whole grains, and organic fruits, nuts, and vegetables.

Tim, who used to skip breakfast, now began his day with

scrambling a couple of high omega-3 eggs in coconut oil and making a large piece of sourdough toast (made from whole wheat flour, not enriched white flour) topped with organic honey fresh from the fields of central California. Lunch was organic chicken or turkey meat on sourdough bread and several handfuls of organic nuts or blueberries. For dinner, he and Suzy would usually grill grass-fed beef or organic chicken purchased at Trader Joe's, an eclectic chain of natural food stores mainly on the West Coast. (I love shopping at Trader Joe's when I'm in California.) They liked to prepare organic vegetables or make a salad from organic produce using olive oil that Tim had pressed. "That way I know the olive oil is unrefined and unprocessed," he said.

Desserts?

"We cut those out," Tim replied.

About halfway through the 7 Weeks of Wellness classes, Tim noticed something—no heartburn, no acid reflux. He wasn't expecting *that* at all: he and Suzy had switched to organic foods as an investment in their future, not to "fix" Tim's heartburn troubles. But eating foods that God created in a form healthy for the body doused his heartburn and dampened his acid reflux.

"I didn't recognize it immediately at the time, but one night I said to Suzy, 'You know what? I haven't had acid reflux since we've been on this new diet.' I felt so much better after I ate, and I felt like my digestive system stabilized. These days, when we're put into a situation where we can't eat healthily like we normally do—like a dinner invitation or a wedding—things have a way of working out. Those one-time mistakes don't result in acid reflux. I'm telling you, this is a great way to go through life."

What a great story Tim Roos has to share! While I can't guarantee that adopting the Great Physician's prescription will eliminate heartburn or acid reflux from your life, I believe the principles behind the seven keys described in the next seven chapters will give you a great shot to make heartburn and acid reflux a distant memory as you unlock your God-given health potential.

Plop, Plop, Fizz, Fizz

The Great Physician's Rx for Heartburn and Acid Reflux is the longest title in this series and, fittingly, quite a mouthful for a book regarding a duo of quintessential American digestive disorders.

Seeking relief for heartburn and acid reflux has, in its own way, become part of the popular culture thanks to zillions of TV and radio advertisements that have successfully drummed the idea into our collective consciousness that "relief is just a swallow away." Some of the most notable—and annoying—television advertising campaigns have transformed a half-dozen over-the-counter antacid products into household names. You would have had to grow up in the backwoods not to recite popular trademarks like Tums, Rolaids, Pepto-Bismol, and Alka-Seltzer off the tip of your tongue.

Alka-Seltzer, the iconic brand known for its cloying "plop, plop, fizz, fizz, oh, what a relief it is" jingle, celebrated seventy-five years of effervescent relief in 2006 by setting a Guinness World Record for the world's largest buffet at the Las Vegas Hilton with 510 potentially heartburn-inducing food items. Patrons passed through a 140-foot-long buffet line, where they could sample:

- 40 different soups (including caramelized onion soup and roasted squash bisque with toasted pepitas)
- 153 cold food offerings (including Waldorf salad and farfalle chicken salad)
- 150 hot food offerings (including BBQ-style beef ribs, Mongolian chicken, cheese quesadillas, crispy buttermilk fried chicken, beef tenderloin tips braised in red wine, tandoori chicken, creamy Israeli couscous, and grilled eggplant)
- 10 carved offerings (including prime rib, honey-glazed ham, and salmon Wellington)
- 5 station offerings (including ginger beef stir fry and hand-rolled chicken soft tacos)
- 152 dessert offerings (including tiramisu, New York–style cheesecake, and crème brûlée tart)

Maybe that March evening would have been a good night to lock up the Alka-Seltzer concession on the Strip, but the truth is that millions of Americans seek relief from overindulgent moments around the clock. According to the latest government statistics, twenty-five million suffer from heartburn daily, while more than sixty million American adults endure occasional occurrences of heartburn. Men and women are affected equally, but the incidence of heartburn increases after age forty.[1] Heartburn is common during pregnancy, probably because of the pressure that the unborn child exerts on the stomach.

Physicians, who say the condition is generally related to what you just ate, lay the blame squarely on Americans' supersized eating habits. There's little doubt that we are devouring more edible fare than ever before—and would gladly eat at the world's largest buffet nightly if given half a chance. The consumption of extra calories is a major reason why we are in the midst of an obesity epidemic and dealing with chronic health problems such as heartburn and acid reflux.

Being heavyset increases pressure on the abdominal area, which in turn amps up the body's production of stomach acids. According to the National Heartburn Alliance, studies have shown that even moderate weight loss can reduce heartburn symptoms.[2] Seventeenth-century British physician Tobias Venner made this observation about the link between being overweight and heartburn: "Men of lean habit of body are commonly a long time healthy, having good appetites and strong stomachs for digestion."[3]

That's not good news for a nation that loves to celebrate every occasion with food—and lots of it. From Saturday nights on the town to festive, all-out holiday dinners, we commemorate life's richest moments with the mouth, tongue, and stomach. The problem is that we are enjoying a bounty of rich, fatty foods six days a week and twice on Sunday while washing everything down with generous amounts of soda, caffeine, and alcohol.

Normally when you eat or drink, the foods and liquids pass through the esophagus, a ten-inch tube that connects the throat to the stomach. Where the stomach and the esophagus meet is the location of a small, one-way valve known as the lower esophageal sphincter. When functioning properly, the lower esophageal sphincter allows everything to pass Go and collect $200 while preventing backward flow. If the lower esophageal sphincter weakens for some reason, as it sometimes does with age, ferocious stomach acids can rise up into the esophagus, resulting in a burning sensation behind the breastbone that lasts from a few minutes to several hours. That's why heartburn has nothing to do with the heart, even though many experience a quite noticeable burning sensation in the cardiovascular area. The inflammation or irritation can feel like dancing flames in the upper chest.

The stomach acids that cause heartburn and acid reflux are also known as hydrochloric acid. To help digest food, the stomach produces about a quart of hydrochloric acid a day to aid in the digestion process. Usually the acid doesn't present a problem because the gastrointestinal tract is coated with a protective mucous lining. When that hydrochloric acid moves up the esophagus, however, watch out. The delicate tissue of the esophagus doesn't have a protective lining as the stomach does, which means that the corrosive nature of the hydrochloric acid produces the burning sensation known around the world as heartburn.

Heartburn is officially identified as pyrosis in medical journals, but it's also medically described as indigestion, acid regurgitation, and sour stomach. Another medical term, nonulcer dyspepsia (NUD), is used to label heartburn troubles not related to an ulcer. Whatever you call it, heartburn and acid reflux are extremely painful conditions that greatly impact one's lifestyle. Heartburn lowers quality of life, while long-term acid reflux can cause scarring and narrowing in the esophagus, which can lead to swallowing difficulties and even prevent food and liquid from reaching the stomach. Other times, the reflux of acid and stomach bile can cause cells in the lining of the esophagus to change and resemble the colon more than the esophagus, which causes a pre-cancerous condition known as Barrett's esophagus.

According to WebMD.com, if one hundred people have heartburn on a regular basis for many years, ten would develop Barrett's esophagus, and one out of those ten would develop esophageal cancer. One out of a hundred may seem like long odds to develop esophageal adenocarcinoma, but this disease has become one of the fastest-growing cancers in the United States, affecting twenty-three persons in one million, up steeply from four in one million in 1975.

Thus, Barrett's esophagus and heartburn are conditions not to be taken lightly.

The Rise of GERD

Acid reflux, the more severe form of indigestion, occurs when sour or bitter-tasting fluids flow up into the mouth or throat after eating. Some say when they lie down, it feels like lava is eroding their tonsils.

When acid reflux hits those pain buttons, it becomes a medical condition known as GERD, an acronym for gastroesophageal reflux disease. Normally, during the act of swallowing, the muscle at the bottom of the esophagus—the lower esophageal sphincter—cooperates by opening up and allowing food into the stomach. With age, stress, or poor physical condition, however, the lower esophageal sphincter can weaken, allowing food and acid to back up the hatch. Left untreated, GERD can lead to ulcers and bleeding of the esophagus as well as increasing the risk of developing cancer of the esophagus.

Don't let friends dismiss GERD as something "in your head" because it's a real disease and a real problem for millions of sufferers. One of those faceless millions is someone very close to me—my father, Dr. Herb Rubin, who has dealt with severe bouts of GERD over the years.

Many heartburn sufferers know that they're setting themselves up for a bad night of sleep when they polish off a late-night pepperoni pizza paired with a hearty merlot. Eating a diet of fatty and fried foods, garlic and onions, spicy foods from the Far East and Mexico, citrus fruits, tomatoes, mint flavorings, and chocolate is tantamount to a declaration of war on the gullet and an invitation for heartburn. Lifestyle decisions, such as smoking cigarettes or drinking alcohol to excess, are contributing factors that weaken or relax the lower esophageal sphincter, which worsens acid reflux. Lying down or kicking back in a recliner has a way of tilting the stomach just so—and allowing stomach acid to spill into the esophagus. Perhaps this is the reason why antacid sales leap by 20 percent the day after the Super Bowl.[4]

Heartburn develops in other ways. The stomach doesn't like stress, which is why you feel "butterflies" in your stomach just before taking a big test or speaking in public. Emotional stress can promote the production of excess stomach acids, prompting all sorts of digestive pain. In addition, the hormones in birth control pills as well as drugs like progesterone, diazepam, and nitroglycerine are known for their causative effects of heartburn.

Food allergies can stimulate histamine release, which stimulates stomach acid secretion. James Breneman, M.D., past president of the American College of Allergists, points out that persistent heartburn from a particular food is a reliable symptom of allergy to that food. Some foods known for causing allergies are dairy products made from cow's milk, wheat, eggs, corn, beef, soy, and some citrus fruits.[5]

CONVENTIONAL TREATMENT

Millions of heartburn sufferers like Tim Roos grin and bear it while reaching for Rolaids. Over-the-counter drugs that neutralize stomach acid are the first line of defense because they're inexpensive and often bring some measure of relief. Familiar brands such as Tums, Maalox, Mylanta, and Milk of Magnesia are antacids that come in tablets or liquids, and they usually consist of one or more of the following ingredients: magnesium, aluminum hydroxide, sodium bicarbonate, or a centuries-old standby known as calcium carbonate. These active compounds buffer the accumulated acids in the stomach.

Antacid tablets are among the best-selling OTC medications in the United States; that's why you're a captive audience for a blitz of primetime TV ads. Drugstore aisles are stacked with the popular name-brand products as well as generic and private labels that urge you to "compare and save."

Right next to the antacids are acid reducers known as H2 blockers. Over-the-counter versions are Zantac 75, Pepcid AC, or Tagamet HB. These drugs block the body's signals to produce acid during digestion. But over time, H2 blockers lose their effectiveness as the body develops a tolerance to this medication.

A more powerful antidote to shutting down the body's production of stomach acids is a class of prescription medications known as proton pump inhibitors (PPIs), which are the most widely prescribed medicines in the United States to treat heartburn, ringing up $12.5 billion in sales in 2004. The top prescription PPIs are Prevacid and Nexium, generating nearly $4 billion *each* in sales at $4 per dose.[6] Talk about a branding coup: I found it interesting that Nexium, which comes in purple pills, can be found on the Internet at www.purplepill.com. (And typing in acidreflux.com will also take you to the Nexium Web site.)

In 2003, the first over-the-counter proton pump inhibitor—Prilosec OTC—was released by Procter & Gamble and within a year became the number one–selling heartburn medicine in the US.[7] The cost per dosage is a far more modest 59 cents. Prilosec OTC's $4 billion in annual sales produces twice the profit generated by every McDonald's, Wendy's, KFC, Taco Bell, and Pizza Hut combined.[8]

Antacids, acid blockers, and proton pump inhibitors have amazing ways to stop the stomach from producing acids, but their use can backfire and lead to *more* instead of less heartburn. Here's how that can happen: while it's generally accepted that heartburn is caused by excess stomach acid, some people who experience severe indigestion actually don't produce enough hydrochloric acid. Fooling the stomach to produce *less* hydrochloric acid robs the digestive system of its ability to digest protein and kill pathogens such as bacteria, viruses, fungi, and parasites. I believe taking meds to shut off the production of stomach acid can be detrimental. When the stomach doesn't have enough hydrochloric acid to properly break down food, the lower esophageal sphincter may weaken and make heartburn and reflux more likely to occur.

Generally speaking, H2 blockers and proton pump inhibitors do what they say they will do—control acid secretion and reduce GERD-like reflux symptoms. The long-term consequences of turning off the production of hydrochloric acid for weeks, months, or years are not known.

What the Doctor Will Say

If you see your family physician, he or she will recommend several lifestyle changes before writing a prescription for a strong acid blocker or proton pump inhibitor (PPI) like Protonex. Lifestyle changes include these:

- eating smaller meals to reduce pressure on the lower esophageal sphincter
- avoiding "trigger foods" that seem to cause heartburn in most folks or eating a large meal soon before bedtime
- quitting smoking and drinking alcohol
- loosening your belt since tightness around your waist puts pressure on the lower abdomen
- not lying down on the couch or waiting at least three hours after eating before you go to bed

- staying slim since being overweight is one of the biggest risk factors for heartburn

- elevating your head by six inches when you sleep by using bricks or blocks to raise the head of your bed

Before seeing a doctor, many people try to relieve their symptoms by changing their eating habits, sitting up straight in couches or chairs, or chewing on antacids. When symptoms become severe and prompt subsequent visits to a doctor, the physician may recommend laparoscopic surgery that involves replacing the stomach to its original position under the diaphragm. The surgeon then wraps and stitches the upper few centimeters of the stomach around the esophagus to prevent reflux from happening again.

ALTERNATIVE MEDICINE

As you would suspect with something as mysterious as the gut, folk remedies and alternative approaches abound for heartburn and acid reflux. Back in Victorian England, an attack of heartburn was met by a stiff upper lip and a shot of brandy. These days, some try to soothe their troubled stomachs with a *digestif,* a French term referring to the consumption of a small crystal glass of high-proof alcohol like cognac, brandy, or whiskey. Fortified wines like port, sherry, or Madeira are digestifs favored by those who don't care for hard spirits.

For those not interested in downing shots after a meal, a no-needle version of acupuncture may offer a new way to battle chronic heartburn, according to a study at the University of Adelaide in Australia. Researchers applied a mild electrical pulse to stimulate an acupressure point on the wrist, which is associated with upper gastrointestinal conditions.[9]

One alternative source, who will go nameless here, even suggested belching as a way to bring relief. I don't think that would fly in my home, but the idea of letting a good burp escape sounds interesting. If you do decide to let one go, just make sure no one is within the distance of a football field since the smell can be nauseating, as Suzy Powell can attest.

A Road Map from Here

Heartburn and acid reflux have a nasty way of defying cure or prevention, but I'm confident that following the Great Physician's prescription for heartburn and acid reflux can alleviate symptoms and nip more serious problems in the bud. The fact that you're reading this book tells me that you (or someone close to you) have complained about acid indigestion and burning feelings in your chest. This is a condition that often strikes in the middle of the night when you're suddenly awakened by a stabbing chest pain. At 1:30 in the morning, you don't have a whole lot of options. Most, like Tim Roos, approach the medicine cabinet with the fervent hope that a few Tums are left in the bottle.

As I mentioned before, I'm not so sure that taking antacids and powerful proton pump inhibitors is the way to go. My approach to dealing with heartburn and acid reflux is based on seven keys to unlock the body's healthy potential that were established in *The Great Physician's Rx for Health and Wellness*:

- Key #1: Eat to Live
- Key #2: Supplement Your Diet with Whole Food Nutritionals, Living Nutrients, and Superfoods
- Key #3: Practice Advanced Hygiene
- Key #4: Condition Your Body with Exercise and Body Therapies
- Key #5: Reduce Toxins in Your Environment
- Key #6: Avoid Deadly Emotions
- Key #7: Live a Life of Prayer and Purpose

Each of these keys can directly support your desire to minimize the effects of digestive stress in your life. But more than that, my main goal for writing *The Great Physician's Rx for Heartburn and Acid Reflux* is to give you a "prevent defense," to use a football term, to prevent heartburn from striking and allow the living God to transform your health as you honor Him physically, mentally, emotionally, and spiritually.

I've certainly had my share of stomach problems, including acid reflux. This will come across sounding like a cliché, but I know a little bit about what you're going through. When I was nineteen years of age back in 1994, I worked as a summer camp counselor following my freshman year at Florida State University. I'll never forget the week I began experiencing nausea, stomach cramps, and horrible digestive problems out of the blue. The constant diarrhea was the worst. I'd be out on the ropes course with the kids when suddenly I'd have this gigantic urge to go. After excusing myself to the other counselors, I'd walk *very quickly*—running was out of the question—to the nearest toilet, which was one of those hole-in-the-floor jobs. It was humiliating!

The relief never lasted long enough. An hour or two later, I'd have to make the same mad dash for the primitive toilets. My energy was sapped by the relentless diarrhea, causing me to lose twenty pounds in just six days. I became one sick puppy and had to leave camp.

That was the start of a two-year health odyssey that began with symptoms of irritable bowel syndrome (IBS) and developed into an inflammatory bowel disease—Crohn's disease. (Irritable bowel syndrome is often mistaken for inflammatory bowel diseases like Crohn's disease or ulcerative colitis, but they're not the same.) During my illness, I suffered from horrible heartburn and was put on prescription-strength Zantac and Pepcid for periods of time.

I tell my story in greater detail in *The Great Physician's Rx for Health and Wellness,* but I did reach a point where I thought I would be better off dying because of searing pain in my gut. I shed pounds like those competing in the reality show *The Biggest Loser.* At my lowest point, I wasn't much more than a stick figure, weighing 104 pounds and resembling a Nazi death camp survivor.

I eventually made a full recovery by employing many of the principles that I share in *The Great Physician's Rx for Heartburn and Acid Reflux.* Today, God has blessed me at age thirty-two with excellent health, and my painful digestive symptoms are in my rearview mirror. Although my stomach troubles were horrible and I wish them upon no one, I also know that God didn't waste my painful experiences. I know I have a deep empathy for those who can't eat a meal in peace without being hit by hideous heartburn.

So does my coauthor, board-certified gastroenterologist Dr. Joseph Brasco, who has treated thousands of patients with heartburn and acid reflux and is highly qualified to help you overcome your digestive problems and regain your health. He knows very well that the nature of heartburn symptoms and painful acid reflux makes these digestive afflictions difficult to discuss with family members, work colleagues, or strangers. When Tim Roos kept his burden concealed as long as possible, he wasn't alone. Those with heartburn and acid reflux prefer to remain in the shadows and suffer in silence.

I don't believe that has to happen. I believe you can get better.

Over the next seven chapters, I will show you how each of the seven keys directly or indirectly relates to heartburn and acid reflux. At the end of this book, I'll give you a seven-day road map to follow. Called the Great Physician's Rx for Heartburn and Acid Reflux Battle Plan, this easy-to-follow lifestyle program will give you the tools you need to make positive changes in your life.

I am convinced that adopting these principles will afford you an excellent chance to greatly reduce the intestinal distress that plagues you or a loved one. I believe each and every one of us has a God-given health potential that can be unlocked only with the right keys. I want to challenge you to incorporate these timeless principles into your life and allow God to transform your health today.

KEY #1

Eat to Live

By their estimation, Michael and Jane Stern have shared more than 72,000 meals over the last three decades, which, according to my math, means an astounding 6.57 meals per day.

Talk about togetherness.

Michael and Jane nosh on three squares a day and then some because they're the authors of *Roadfood* and *Two for the Road: Our Love Affair with American Food.* Their books have been described as glove-box bibles for chain-weary travelers seeking authentic barbecue or cheese-topped apple pie à la mode just like Grandma used to make.

From their home base in Connecticut, the Sterns crisscross the country one hundred days a year in search of the perfect diner. They've logged more than three million miles on America's two-lane highways, dropping in at roadside cafes and small town restaurants to sample flapjacks, *huevos grande,* Philly cheesesteaks, clam pizza, chili dogs, Cajun gumbo, garlic-and-shrimp fettuccini, barbecue brisket, Maine lobster, and chicken fried steak. The Sterns love discovering—and writing about—little-known regional specialties like Grape-Nuts pudding, fried tripe, and pig's ear. In the midst of their on-the-road research, this husband-and-wife team somehow manages to eat an average of twelve meals per day: four breakfasts, four lunches, and four dinners. They don't count the afternoon stops for an ice cream treat.

1

As the Sterns are quick to say, it's a tough job, but some-body's got to do it. Michael and Jane wake up before dawn so that they're ready for the 6:00 a.m. opening of the next greasy spoon on their list. Once their first Belgian waffle is under their belts, it's on to the next roadside diner for a Denver omelet and hash browns. "We can eat just about anyone under the table, so the first few breakfasts of the day are no problem at all," they boast in *Two for the Road*.

I'm expecting the Sterns to land an endorsement deal for Alka-Seltzer or Pepto-Bismol any day now because I don't see how you can eat that much processed, sweet-sauced, sugar-coated, candied, sticky, salty, barbecued, battered, and fried food without developing a major tummy ache. The Sterns' success—they sell tons of books and are regularly featured on NPR's *The Splendid Table* radio show—is testimony to the fact that we've become a country that loves inexpensive deep-fried, greasy food that's high in calories, high in fat, high in sugar, and—in most people's minds—high in taste. Taste trumps health, no matter how many calories or fat grams the food contains.

In my opinion, it's not hard to conclude that this type of nutritional sustenance is an eight-lane freeway to poor health. Don't folks know that they're steering themselves the wrong direction on a one-way street? Aren't they aware that they're set-ting themselves up for bouts of painful heartburn or acid reflux by making poor choices in what they eat?

I guess not. In fact, I'm convinced that too many people coast through life without thinking two seconds about the significance of what they eat or the quantities they consume. Part of the blame can be laid at the feet of modern media, which broadcasts alluring and effective commercials for bacon-topped cheeseburgers on ciabatta buns and the newest deep-dish, stuffed-crust, cheeselover, full-house, quadruple-meat, super-deluxe pizza. On the print side, you can stroll into a supersized bookstore and scrutinize hundreds of titles—many containing conflicting information—about how to lose weight, eat right, and live a long, healthy life. I'm afraid that many of the latest health books come and go because people aren't looking at a single, constant source of good nutrition and healthy living—the Bible.

I believe we can look to Scripture to be reminded about what God created for food. My friend Rex Russell, M.D., compiled a comprehensive list of foods created by God in his book *What the Bible Says About Healthy Living.* I've listed them here, along with the scriptural references. As you scan this list, ask yourself how many people order these foods at a roadside diner:

- almonds (Gen. 43:11)
- barley (Judg. 7:13)
- beans (Ezek. 4:9)
- bread (1 Sam. 17:17)
- broth (Judg. 6:19)
- cakes (2 Sam. 13:8 [NKJV], and probably not the kind with frosting)
- cheese (Job 10:10)
- cucumbers, onions, leeks, melons, and garlic (Num. 11:5)

- curds of cow's milk (Deut. 32:14)
- figs (Num. 13:23)
- fish (Matt. 7:10)
- fowl (1 Kings 4:23)
- fruit (2 Sam. 16:2)
- game (Gen. 25:28)
- goat's milk (Prov. 27:27)
- grain (Ruth 2:14)
- grapes (Deut. 23:24)
- grasshoppers, locusts, and crickets (Lev. 11:22)
- herbs (Exod. 12:8)
- honey (Isa. 7:15) and wild honey (Ps. 19:10)
- lentils (Gen. 25:34)
- meal (Matt. 13:33 KJV)
- pistachio nuts (Gen. 43:11)
- oil (Prov. 21:17)
- olives (Deut. 28:40)
- pomegranates (Num. 13:23)
- quail (Num. 11:32)
- raisins (2 Sam. 16:1)
- salt (Job 6:6)
- sheep (Deut. 14:4)
- sheep's milk (Deut. 32:14)
- spices (Gen. 43:11)

- veal (Gen. 18:7–8)

- vegetables (Prov. 15:17)

- vinegar (Num. 6:3)[1]

My guess is that the Sterns don't find too many of these foods when they're doing their road warrior thing. What about you? Are any of these staples in your diet? Do you have to think hard to remember the last time you peeled a fresh orange, scooped up a handful of dates, or supped on lentil soup? These listed foods are nutritional gold mines and contain no refined or processed carbohydrates, no trans-fatty acids, and no artificial sweeteners. Since God has given us a bountiful harvest of natural foods to eat, it would take several pages to describe all the fantastic fruits and vibrant vegetables available from His garden.

For this reason, *The Great Physician's Rx for Heartburn and Acid Reflux* relies heavily on my first key, "Eat to Live," which can be summed up by this pair of statements:

1. Eat what God created for food.
2. Eat food in a form that is healthy for the body.

If you're following the standard American diet—a Danish pastry or bowl of sugar-frosted cereal for breakfast; a rainbow-sprinkled doughnut for a midmorning snack; a processed turkey and ham sandwich, barbecue-flavored potato chips, and a diet soft drink for lunch; a candy bar for an afternoon snack; a take-out pepperoni pizza and garlic bread for dinner; and chocolate chip ice cream for dessert—then you better get used to popping those Tums because your heartburn and acid reflux aren't going away anytime soon.

Your better course would be taking the first key of the Great Physician's prescription to heart. Not only would "Eat to Live" do you a world of good, but following these two vital concepts will also give you a great shot to douse heartburn and put you on the road toward living a healthy, vibrant life. "Let food be thy medicine; thy medicine shall be thy food," said Hippocrates, the ancient Greek physician and father of medicine.

Many heartburn sufferers, after being beaten down by this affliction and seeking medical attention, follow their doctors' recommendations and resign themselves to a dull diet of oatmeal, egg whites, baked potatoes, broccoli, skinless chicken breast without a scent of seasoning, and fat-free—and taste-free—dairy products. I don't think you're doomed to eat bland or even non-acidic foods when you're dealing with chronic indigestion or acid reflux. In fact, some of the best foods you can consume are foods that are acidic by nature. Here's what I mean.

Foods can be generally classified into acid-forming and alkaline-forming foods, which is calculated when the foods are burned and their ash is measured. Foods have a pH value range from 0 (most acidic) to 14 (most alkaline). A common misconception is that if a food tastes acidic, it must form acid in the stomach, but that's not always the case when it comes to heartburn. For instance, acidic lemons, limes, and apple cider vinegar are actually highly alkaline forming due to their mineral content. In fact, the aforementioned are examples of foods or liquids that you could consume because they can dilute stomach acid and reduce pain.

Other foods that you want to make sure you're eating are fruits and vegetables with edible skins, whole grains, nuts, seeds, and beans. These high-fiber foods—made up of indigestible remnants of plant cells—have little potential to cause heartburn because they move through the digestive system quickly prior to elimination from the body. When food lingers too long in the stomach, however, that can cause problems like bacterial overgrowth as stomach acids work overtime. Eating fiber-rich foods will keep things moving and could protect you from the more serious affliction of gastroesophageal reflux disease (GERD). In 2005, researchers at the Houston Veterans Affairs Medical Center performed a study showing that high-fiber diets were protective against GERD, regardless of one's body weight.[2]

I also recommend the consumption of naturally fermented or cultured foods that contain probiotics and enzymes, which are part of the Great Physician's Rx for Heartburn and Acid Reflux Battle Plan in the back of this book. In the meantime, though, we need to talk about everything you put into your mouth since that's a major key to dealing with heartburn. Every time you take a bite of food, you're sending a protein, a fat, or a carbohydrate into your gullet. Let's take a closer look at these macronutrients.

THE FIRST WORD ON PROTEINS

Proteins, one of the basic components of foods, are the essential building blocks of the body and involved in the function of every living cell, including those parked in the digestive tract.

One of protein's main tasks is to provide specific nutrient material to grow and repair cells.

All proteins are combinations of twenty-two amino acids, which build and maintain the body's organs, including the heart, as well as the muscles and nerves, to name a few important duties. Your body, however, cannot produce all twenty-two amino acids that you need to live a robust life. Scientists have discovered that eight essential amino acids are missing, meaning that they must come from sources outside the body. I know the following fact drives vegetarians and vegans crazy, but animal protein—chicken, beef, lamb, dairy, eggs, and so forth—is the *only* complete protein source providing the Big Eight amino acids in the right quantities and ratios.

Tom Cowan, M.D., a San Francisco physician in private practice, had an interesting take on this in the quarterly magazine of the Weston A. Price Foundation, founded on the principles taught by a man I deeply respect, Weston A. Price. (Price was a Cleveland dentist who became a pioneer in urging people to stop eating processed foods.) At any rate, Dr. Cowan wrote that when it comes to heartburn, nearly everyone accepts the fact that the burning sensation is caused by excess stomach acid. Since protein foods are responsible for the stomach cells to produce acid, conventional medical advice is straightforward for heartburn therapy: eat less protein (i.e., fatty hamburgers) so that less acid will be produced.

Dr. Cowan said there's another theory regarding heartburn, which is that the stomach naturally produces acid in response to eating *any* food, not just a protein like chicken or steak. This is because stomach acid kills invading microorganisms present in the food we eat, protecting us from infections occurring in the gastrointestinal tract. "Furthermore, the very group of people who lacks stomach acid, that is the elderly, is the group that most suffers from GERD," Dr. Cowan wrote. "So in this case, the solution is not to inhibit production by eating less protein, but rather to increase protein—and fat—consumption so as to give the acid something to do, which is to digest the protein."[3]

I don't believe that you have to give up red meat when you have heartburn and acid reflux *if* you're served the leanest, healthiest sources of animal protein available, which come from organically raised cattle, sheep, goats, buffalo, and venison—animals that graze on pastureland grasses. Lean grass-fed beef is lower in calories and doesn't contain as much fat as grain-fed beef.

As mentioned before, everyone agrees chicken and fish are excellent sources of protein for those with heartburn problems. That's good news because I'm a huge fan of free-range chicken and fish caught from lakes, streambeds, or ocean depths. Fish with scales and fins, caught in the wild, contain healthy fats, vitamins, and minerals, and provide all the essential amino acids. Wild fish, which is nutritionally far superior to farm-raised, should be consumed liberally.

The Skinny on Fats

A century ago, he was the Dr. Atkins of his time. When Bertram Sippy, a Chicago physician, treated patients with gastrointestinal distress back in the early 1900s, he required them to drink small amounts of milk and light cream to counteract stomach acids. No fruits and vegetables. Adherents called it the "Sippy Diet," and doctors used it to treat heartburn until the 1970s when it was universally shelved.[4]

These days the conventional wisdom is that the consumption of high-fat foods like milk and cream is double trouble since these fatty foods need more time to break down in the stomach, which prolongs the time that acid reflux can occur. Regular full-fat milk and cheese are held up as examples of foods that exacerbate heartburn conditions. This directive sums up today's by-the-medical-book advice: when dealing with heartburn, shun high-fat foods and increase fiber.

I'm all for increasing fiber, but I part ways with those who declare certain foods containing what I consider to be healthy fats off limits. You see, the problem with the standard American diet is that people eat too many of the wrong foods containing the wrong fats and not enough of the right foods with the right fats. On top of that, there's a lot of confusion about fats in this world because we hear how bad they are when, in fact, fats are essential because they regulate insulin levels and trigger enzymes that convert food into energy.

Eating healthy fats can have a protective effect against many diseases, including the *real* heartburn—cardiovascular disease. I'm referring to foods loaded with the following:

- polyunsaturated fats (high in omega-3 fatty acids)
- monounsaturated (omega-9) fatty acids
- conjugated linoleic acid (CLA)

- key omega-6 fats, such as gamma-linolenic acid (GLA)
- healthy saturated fats containing short- and medium-chain fatty acids, such as butter and coconut oil

It's worth noting again that these good fats are found in a wide range of foods, including salmon, cod-liver oil, lamb, goat meat, and high omega-3 eggs, dairy products derived from goat's milk, sheep's milk, cow's milk and butter from grass-fed animals, flaxseeds, walnuts, olives, macadamia nuts, and avocados. People are often shocked to hear me say this, but this is why I say butter is better for you than margarine. Organically produced butter is loaded with healthy fatty acids such as short-chain saturated fatty acids, which supply energy to the body and aid in the regeneration of the digestive tract. Margarine, on the other hand, is a man-made, congealed conglomeration of chemicals and hydrogenated liquid vegetable oils.

Fats and oils created by God, as you would expect, are fats you want to include in your diet. The top two on my list are extra virgin coconut and olive oils, which are beneficial to the body and can aid metabolism. I urge you to cook with extra virgin coconut oil, which is a near miracle food that few people have ever heard of.

THE TRUTH ABOUT CARBOHYDRATES

Of the different macronutrients—proteins, fats, and carbohydrates—carbohydrates have the biggest effect on gastrointestinal health. Carbohydrates, especially those from refined sources, are high in hard-to-digest components such as complex sugars, phytates, and gluten.

By definition, carbohydrates are the sugars and starches contained in plant foods. Sugars and starches, like fats, are not bad for you, but the problem for those fighting heartburn is that the standard American diet includes way too many foods containing these refined carbohydrates. While health-care providers rightfully recommend that you avoid eating sugar unnecessarily, that's easier said than done. Sugar and its sweet relatives—high fructose corn syrup, sucrose, molasses, and maple syrup—are among the first ingredients listed in staples such as cereals, breads, buns, pastries, doughnuts, cookies, ketchup, and ice cream. Tim Roos thought he was eating well until he realized that the cereals, breads, and buns in his kitchen were processed foods made from refined sources.

The Great Physician's prescription for heartburn and acid reflux calls for eating healthy proteins, healthy fats, and lower amounts of carbohydrates (sugars and starches). Restricting the consumption of carbohydrates and wisely choosing your carbs should result in an improvement in intestinal flora, or microorganisms. Few people have heard of intestinal flora or are aware that there are trillions of cells in the human body but even more microbial cells in the large intestine in the form of intestinal flora. The body permits these friendly bacteria and yeasts to live in the intestinal tract because they are a line of defense against disease-causing bacteria, viruses, toxins, and parasites.

The carbohydrates you want to consume are low glycemic, high nutrient, and low sugar. These would be most high-fiber fruits (especially berries), vegetables, nuts, seeds, and some legumes, plus a small amount of whole grain products (sprouted, soaked, or sour-leavened), which are always better than refined carbohydrates that have been stripped of their vital fiber, essential fatty acids, vitamins, and mineral components.

How Well Are You Chewing Your Food?

When you grab a forkful of pasta or bite into a delicious apple, you begin chewing and swallowing your food, an elementary process that you've probably taken for granted since your mother spoon-fed you applesauce in a high chair.

A little biology lesson: after you swallow, the food enters your esophagus, the ten-inch-long muscular tube that leads to the stomach. How long the food spends in the esophagus depends on how well it was chewed. Food that has been chewed well—properly masticated, as they say in jolly old England—makes the journey in just seven seconds. Food that's dry or not properly chewed can take a full minute to wend its way through the esophagus, which is not good for the delicate tissues lining this tube between the throat and the stomach. Improperly chewed food that reaches the stomach takes longer to digest, which creates acute, temporary stress on the entire gastrointestinal process.

Eating quickly and not chewing your food properly also put too much pressure on the lower esophageal sphincter, which could cause the sphincter muscle to weaken and allow acid from the stomach to invade the esophagus. Bingo . . . a classic case of heartburn.

Chewing your food well can do a lot for relieving heartburn pains. Chewing food properly allows enzymes in your saliva to turn the food into a near liquid form before swallowing. The mucus in saliva adheres to food, making it slippery so that the lubricated food can shimmy down the esophagus like a fireman sliding down a slick pole to answer an emergency call. The act of working your jaw also sends a neurological message to your stomach and pancreas to increase acid and digestive enzyme production because food's on the way.

Chances are that you haven't heard of "The Great Masticator," which was the moniker given to Horace Fletcher, a British nutritionist at the turn of the last century. A raconteur, world traveler, millionaire businessman, amateur painter, speaker, and author, Fletcher tirelessly promoted his theory of good chewing: he recommended that food be chewed thirty-two times—which works the jaw one hundred times per minute—before being swallowed. "Nature will castigate those who don't masticate," he warned. Followers of "Fletcherism," as his doctrine became known, included industrialist John D. Rockefeller and authors Upton Sinclair and Henry James.

I know that chewing your food that many times seems like an arduous task, but masticating your food thoroughly—especially foods high in carbohydrates—can enhance the digestive process and reduce postmeal bloating. Chewing slowly and thoroughly can also help maintain a healthy weight as you allow your brain to register the amount of food you are consuming. Eating too fast creates large pieces of food difficult for digestive enzymes to handle, causing heartburn. If you're chomping on hamburgers or sandwiches while you drive, then you're setting yourself up for gastric distress and a bout of heartburn and burping.

I rarely eat and drive at the same time, but more important, I've become a much better "chewer." In fact, if you were to dine with me sometime, you'd be surprised at how long I take to chew my food. It has taken some effort on my part to reprogram the way I eat, yet I know that a conscious effort to chew food slowly ensures that plenty of digestive juices are added to the food as it begins to wind through the digestive tract.

The Top Healing Foods

I've been talking in general terms about nutritional recommendations, but now I would like to be more specific. Let's take a closer look at what you should eat when it comes to keeping heartburn at bay:

1. Chicken soup. Stop scratching your head. Homemade chicken soup—I'm talking about the kind made from homemade chicken stock with fresh, organic ingredients—is easy to digest and contains gelatin, which has potentially enormous benefits for heartburn sufferers.

I know that when most people hear the word *gelatin*, they're thinking about Jell-O, a bland, artificially flavored dessert that's synonymous with retirement home dinners and kids' birthday parties. The gelatin I'm referring to is a colorless, odorless, and flavorless mixture of proteins that's obtained from boiling animals' bones and connective tissues in water.

The Weston A. Price Foundation, after conducting thorough research, states that a substantial body of evidence suggests that gelatin has great value in health and digestion. Kaayla T. Daniel, writing on the Weston A. Price Web site, declared, "Meats found in soup and pot roasts—cooked with bones for a long time in a liquid to which a touch of vinegar has been added—are easier to digest than quickly cooked steaks and chops."[5] Properly prepared, meat stocks are extremely nutritious, containing the minerals of bones, cartilage, marrow, and vegetables that supply the body with hydrophilic colloids, which attract digestive juices for rapid and effective digestion.

Ms. Daniel also quoted the research of Francis Pottenger, M.D., who spent years researching gelatin. "Gelatin may be used in conjunction with almost any diet that the clinician feels is indicated," said Dr. Pottenger. "Its colloidal properties aid the digestion of any foods which cause the patient to suffer from 'sour stomach.' Even foods to which individuals may be definitely sensitive, as proven by the leucopenic index and elimination diets, frequently may be tolerated with slight discomfort or none at all if gelatin is made part of the diet."[6]

It doesn't surprise me that chicken soup is good for the soul and for the stomach. I've had a soft spot for chicken soup ever since Mom and Grandma Rose nursed me back to health with steaming bowls of this hearty meal a dozen years ago. The recuperative effects of chicken soup date as far back as the twelfth century when the Jewish physician and philosopher Moses Maimonides recommended its use for the treatment of respiratory infections.

My wife, Nicki, who's a wonderful cook, and I have come up with an excellent recipe that we call tongue-in-cheek "Heartburn-Bustin' Chicken Soup." This recipe was inspired by Sally Fallon, author of *Nourishing Traditions*. You definitely should go to the trouble to add chicken feet to this recipe, which Jewish folklore considers the secret to a successful broth:

Heartburn-Bustin' Chicken Soup

Ingredients:

    1 whole chicken (free range, pastured, or organic chicken)
    2–4 chicken feet (optional)
    3–4 quarts filtered water
    1 tablespoon raw apple cider vinegar
    4 medium-sized onions, coarsely chopped
    8 carrots, peeled and coarsely chopped
    6 celery stalks, coarsely chopped
    2–4 zucchinis, chopped

4–6 tablespoons extra virgin coconut oil

1 bunch parsley

5 garlic cloves (optional for the heartburn sufferer)

4 inches grated ginger

2–4 tablespoons Celtic Sea Salt

1/4–1/2 teaspoon cayenne pepper (optional for the heartburn sufferer)

Directions:

If you are using a whole chicken, remove fat glands and the gizzards from the cavity. By all means, use chicken feet if you can find them. Place chicken or chicken pieces in a large stainless steel pot with the water, vinegar, and all vegetables except parsley. Let stand for 10 minutes before heating. Bring to a boil and remove scum that rises to the top. Cover and cook for 12 to 24 hours. The longer you cook the stock, the more healing it will be. About 15 minutes before finishing the stock, add the parsley. This will impart additional mineral ions to the broth.

Remove from heat, and take out the chicken and the chicken feet. Let it cool and remove chicken meat from the carcass, discarding the bones and the feet. Drop the meat back into the soup and combine with the other ingredients.

2. Wild-caught fish. Eating wild-caught fish is a winning strategy for heartburn. For those who say you should stay away from "fatty" foods like the flesh of fish, my reply is, "Hogwash." Fish, especially those caught in the wild, are a rich source of omega-3 fats, protein, potassium, vitamins, and minerals. The essential fatty acids play a crucial role in the body's chemistry, constituting at least 50 percent of all cell membranes, building up the health of our bones, enhancing the immune system, protecting the liver from alcohol and other toxins, and guarding against harmful microorganisms in the digestive tract.

Choose fresh salmon and other fish from your local fish market or health food store that is labeled Alaskan or wild-caught. Wild-caught fish is an absolutely incredible food and should be consumed liberally.

3. Fruits and vegetables. For the most part, fruits and vegetables are alkaline forming and have little potential to cause heartburn. Most fruits and veggies are high in potassium and other minerals, which are great for digestion. Don't deep-fry your vegetables in batter; that's an unhealthy way to prepare vegetables even if you've never experienced heartburn.

Highly alkalizing fruits are peaches, apricots, grapes, bananas, raisins, prunes, coconuts, melons, pears, figs, dates, avocados, and apples.

Highly alkalizing vegetables are okra, squash, green beans, peppers, lima beans, mushrooms, carrots, corn, lettuce, cucumbers, sweet peas, beets, parsley, and potatoes.

Of course, you'll be miles ahead if you purchase organic foods, and it makes shopping easier that major supermarket chains—even Wal-Mart—are stocking more and more organic fruits and vegetables in their produce departments. Sure, you'll pay anywhere from 10 to 100 percent more, but what kind of price tag can you put on relieving heavy heartburn or painful acid reflux?

4. Cultured dairy products from goats, cows, and sheep. Two items that doctors are quick to cross off your shopping list are full-fat cow's milk and yogurt, since the calcium and protein in these dairy products stimulate the production of more acid. Physicians lump the saturated fats in dairy products in the same category as red meat, implicating the fat intake as a key factor behind heartburn and acid reflux. Thus, doctors recommend that you should not eat full-fat dairy products when heartburn is a regular nighttime visitor. They counsel shopping for low-fat versions of dairy products, like 2 percent or skim milk or low-fat yogurt.

Even though some believe that skim and low-fat dairy products are easier on the stomach, they aren't healthy to consume. When I speak before audiences, I joke that I've never heard of a milking cow or goat producing 2 percent or skim milk. On a more serious note, fat-free and reduced-fat dairy products are less nutritious, even *less* digestible, and can cause allergies, which is one of the top unsuspected causes of gastrointestinal problems. I think a much better approach to heartburn is purchasing dairy products derived from goat's milk and sheep's milk, although you could try dairy products from organic or grass-fed cows to see if they agree with your tumultuous tummy.

The reason I prefer goat's milk and goat's cheese lies in the structure of the goat's milk: its fat and protein molecules are tiny in size, which allows for rapid absorption in the digestive tract. Milk fat also contains a number of bioactive components, including conjugated linoleic acid (CLA).

Goat's milk contains a little less lactose and is filled with vitamins, enzymes, and protein. Although it does have a more pungent smell and taste than cow's milk, you should be aware that outside the United States, 65 percent of the world's population drinks goat's milk—and considers the taste to be delicious. Goat's cheese is a wonderful food to add to your salads.

I also highly recommend eating fermented dairy products such as yogurt, kefir, hard cheeses, cultured cream cheese, cottage cheese, and cultured cream. Those who are lactose-intolerant can often stomach fermented dairy products because they contain little or no residual lactose, which is the type of sugar in milk that many find hard to digest.

5. Apple cider vinegar. You may have noticed that I included apple cider vinegar as an ingredient for the Heartburn-Bustin' Chicken Soup recipe, and you'll see that I recommend it daily in the Great Physician's Rx for Heartburn and Acid Reflux Battle Plan. There was a reason for that. I believe apple cider vinegar is an important substance to drink when you have heartburn and acid reflux.

Apple cider vinegar is made from squeezed liquid of crushed apples. Sugar and yeast are added to the liquid to start the fermentation process, which turns the sugar into alcohol. During a second round of fermentation, the alcohol is converted by acetic acid-forming bacteria into vinegar. The acetic acid gives vinegar its sour taste, as well as its minerals: potassium, phosphorus, calcium, magnesium, natural silicon, pectin, malic acid, and tartaric acids, which help the body maintain its vital acid-alkaline balance. The acidity in apple cider vinegar helps the body rebalance its acid level, which is important as the body tries to find its equilibrium while digesting food. The icky taste hasn't stopped aficionados from singing the praises of apple cider vinegar, or ACV for short.

The "Johnny Appleseed" of apple cider vinegar is a Vermont physician, D. C. Jarvis, M.D., who injected the lore of folk medicine into his practice. His book, *Folk Medicine,* has sold more than three million copies over the last fifty years. Apple cider vinegar will destroy pathogenic bacteria in your digestive tract, he says.

Remember: don't drink apple cider vinegar unless it is well diluted. I recommend two teaspoons of ACV and two teaspoons of honey mixed in eight to twelve ounces of warm water; otherwise, you'll be puckering your lips and shaking your head from tartness of the first sip.

6. Water. Fereydoon Batmanghelidj, M.D., author of *Your Body's Many Cries for Water,* contends that heartburn is a signal from the body that it's not getting enough water. Unless you start drinking more water, you're setting yourself up for more bothersome conditions such as dyspeptic pain or a peptic ulcer.

"Because we do not recognize heartburn as a signal of body thirst, its significance is not understood until an ulcer develops," Dr. Batmanghelidj said. "Everyone should be alert to heartburn as a major thirst pain of the body."[7]

Dr. Batmanghelidj explained that when we drink a glass of water, this life-giving resource is immediately passed into the digestive system, where it is quickly absorbed by the body. Water flowing through the mucous layer of the stomach brings about the expansion and thickening of this protective layer of the stomach. When you're dehydrated, however, the mucous barrier is rendered ineffective as a buffer against stomach acids. As for the lower esophageal sphincter, Dr. Batmanghelidj believes that this "gate" between the esophagus and the stomach becomes lax from chronic dehydration.

The solution is simple: drink more water. I realize this is a shocking conclusion, but the conscious mind has a problem with recognizing the body's water needs. "Full and adequate hydration of the body depends on the sharpness of its thirst perception," Dr. Batmanghelidj wrote. "Unfortunately, as it ages, the body gradually loses its ability to recognize its dehydration. Elderly people can become chronically dehydrated, even if there is plenty of drinking water available, because they fail to recognize their extreme thirst."[8]

Before sitting down for a meal, Dr. Batmanghelidj recommends drinking an ample amount of water—a full glass or two— a half hour before eating. By this action, the cells will become well hydrated when the body begins the digestion process and won't need to tap into water held inside the cells lining the blood vessels.

Throughout the rest of the day, you should drink a minimum of eight glasses of water to stay hydrated. Sure, you'll go to the bathroom more often, but is that so bad? Drinking plenty of water is not only healthy for the body, but it's a key part of the Great Physician's Rx for Heartburn and Acid Reflux Battle Plan (see page 75), so keep a water bottle close by and drink water before, during, and in between meals.

I take hydration seriously even though I don't have heartburn. I set a forty-eight-ounce bottle of water on my office desk as a reminder to keep putting fluids into my system. My record for drinking water is one and one-quarter gallons of water in a day during a fast, but I won't reveal how many trips I made to the bathroom that day!

Okay, so you'll treble your steps to the lavatory by consciously drinking more water, but you'll be giving your digestive system the "lubrication" it needs to keep everything moving . . . and not backing up and causing heartburn.

7. Raw organic honey. If apple cider vinegar is too tart for your taste, then consider sweet honey, which has gained a following for its treatment of heartburn symptoms and soothing protection of the esophagus. Simply lick one teaspoon of raw organic honey or spread a spoonful on a small piece of bread or fruit twenty minutes before breakfast, lunch, dinner, or bedtime. Do not drink any liquids during these twenty minutes to allow the honey to stay as concentrated as possible.

WHAT NOT TO EAT: "THE DIRTY DOZEN"

No matter what your heartburn problems are, the following foods—which I call "The Dirty Dozen"—should never find a way onto your plate or into your hands. Some I've already discussed elsewhere in this chapter, while the rest are presented here with a short commentary:

1. Processed meat and pork products. These meats top my list because they are staples in the standard American diet and extremely unhealthy. You must steer clear of breakfast links, bacon, lunchmeats, ham, bratwurst, and other sausages because they introduce pathogenic organisms and toxins into the bloodstream that compromise digestion. These processed meats contain additives like nitrates that were introduced during the curing process. Nitrates can convert into nitrite, which can form into nitrosamines, a powerful cancer-causing chemical.

Many processed meats—including pepperoni, salami, and hot dogs—are made from pork products. In all of my previous books, I've consistently pointed out that pork—America's "other white meat"—should be avoided because pigs were called "unclean" and "detestable" in Leviticus and Exodus. God created pigs as scavengers—animals that survive just fine on any farm slop or water swill tossed their way. Pigs have a simple stomach arrangement: whatever a pig eats goes down the hatch, straight into the stomach, and out the back door in four hours maximum. They'll even eat their own excrement, if hungry enough.

Even if you decide to keep eating commercial beef instead of the organic version, I absolutely urge you to stop eating pork. Read Leviticus 11 and Deuteronomy 14 to learn what God said about eating clean versus unclean animals, where Hebrew words used to describe "unclean meats" can be translated as "foul" and "putrid," the same terms the Bible uses to describe human waste.

Eating unclean foods fouls the body and may lead to increases in stomach distress, heart disease, and cancer by introducing toxins into the bloodstream. God declared these meats unclean because He understands the ramifications of eating them, and you should as well.

2. Shellfish and fish without fins and scales, such as catfish, shark, and eel. Shellfish and fish without fins and scales, are also described in Leviticus 11 and Deuteronomy 14 as "unclean meats." God called hard-shelled crustaceans such as lobster, crabs, shrimp, and clams unclean because they are "bottom feeders," content to sustain themselves on excrement from other fish. To be sure, this purifies water but does nothing for the health of their flesh—or yours, if you eat them.

Am I saying au revoir and sayonara to lobster thermidor and shrimp tempura? You can bet your scampi.

3. Hydrogenated oils. Hydrogenated fats and partially hydrogenated fats are found in practically every processed food, from Dunkin' Donuts to Wonder Bread, from Ding Dongs to Dove Bars. Most of the oils used in households today—soybean, safflower, cottonseed, and corn—are partially hydrogenated oils, which, by definition, are liquid fats that have been injected with hydrogen gas at high temperatures under high pressure to make them solid at room temperature.

Hydrogenation increases shelf life and gives flavor stability to foods, but it also produces unsaturated trans-fatty acids, also known as trans fats. Mark my words: trans fats are terribly unhealthy for the body and a difficult-to-digest substance. For years, you couldn't find out how much trans fat was in the food you're eating, but that changed in 2006 with the introduction of new nutrition facts labels stating the amount of trans fat in that particular food. I welcome this long-overdue change in food labeling, although I don't see the sales of processed foods declining.

Be aware that the hydrogenated or partially hydrogenated fats in processed foods—from commercial cakes, pastries, and desserts to just about every wrapped-in-plastic item sold in a neighborhood convenience store—are hard on the stomach and stay in the body a long time, causing more digestive mischief. The processing process—try saying that ten times in a row—inhibits or removes the natural enzymes that cause foods to spoil, but that impedes our intestinal enzymes from digesting the nutrients out of the foods, too.

If you can hop off the junk food bandwagon and leave all those hydrogenated oils behind, your stomach will thank you.

4. Artificial sweeteners. I find it highly ironic that aspartame—the artificial sweetener found in NutraSweet and Equal—was originally conceived as a drug to treat peptic ulcers. Back in 1965, a chemist named James Schlatter, working for G. D. Searle & Company on anti-ulcer formulations, happened to lick his finger, which had accidentally become contaminated with aspartame. He tasted a sweet, attractive flavor, albeit highly concentrated, of course.

An artificial sweetener was serendipitously born, but it took G. D. Searle more than fifteen years for aspartame to be approved by the US Food and Drug Administration because of a nasty little problem—lab rats got cancer. The chemical additive was finally approved for dry goods in 1981 and carbonated beverages in 1983. But here's Irony No. 2: aspartame is also an ingredient in several H2-blocking heartburn and ulcer-treating medications, including Pepcid AC and Zantac, according to the Mayo Clinic Web site.

My friend Dr. Joe Mercola, of the influential Mercola.com Web site, says that aspartame accounts for more than 75 percent of the adverse reactions to food additives reported to the FDA. We're talking about headaches, dizziness, numbness, nausea, and other digestive difficulties. The Internet is filled with bloggers complaining about how aspartame caused their heartburn, so there's anecdotal evidence as well. I would hope that aspartame, saccharin (Sweet 'N Low), and sucralose (Splenda) have been banished from your home as well. In my opinion, these blue, pink, and yellow packets are questionable compounds that don't deserve a place in your cupboard or your cup of coffee.

5. White flour. After wheat is harvested, the wheat stalks are trucked to flour mills and rinsed with various chemical bleaches that sound like a vocabulary test from high school biology class: nitrogen oxide, chlorine, chloride, nitrosyl, and benzoyl peroxide. The result is that half of the healthy fatty acids are lost in the milling process, as well as the wheat germ and bran, which contain vitamins and fiber. By removing most of the naturally occurring nutrients and adding chemicals and a few isolated and synthetic vitamins and minerals, we've managed to take a healthy food that's been on families' tables for centuries—usually in the form of bread, pasta, or baked goods—and turn it into one of the most highly allergenic, difficult-to-digest substances.

"Enriched" or unbleached flour contains hard-to-digest starches that cause indigestion and bad bacterial and yeast overgrowth. The healthier alternative is eating whole wheat bread made from unprocessed whole grain flour.

6. White sugar. Here's another food that promotes heartburn and bacterial and yeast overgrowth. Sugar comes in so many forms that it's hard to keep track of the names used for it these days. If the food label uses descriptions like corn syrup, high fructose corn syrup, sucrose, corn sweeteners, sorghum syrup, and/or fruit juice concentrate, you're essentially eating sugar.

Sugar is the first ingredient on a bar of chocolate. I hate to be the bearer of bad news for chocolate lovers out there, but chocolate has been clinically shown to relax the lower esophageal sphincter, which allows stomach acids to squirt up into the esophagus, according to a medical study released by the Bowman Gray School of Medicine at Wake Forest University.[9]

So the moral of the story: eat less sugar and ditch the chocolate. Peppermint, spearmint, and other mints must be crossed off your list as well since many report having acid reflux problems after eating mints.

7. Soft drinks. If you're a member of the Pepsi generation, carbonated soft drinks are among the strongest predictors of nighttime heartburn, according to a 2005 study released by the University of Arizona College of Medicine.[10] This doesn't surprise me since soft drinks are nothing more than liquefied sugar with bubbles. A twelve-ounce cola is the equivalent of eating nearly nine teaspoons of sugar. Popular soft drinks also contain chemicals that cause the body to become more acidic, which is not a great feeling for the stomach and heartburn sufferers.

8. Pasteurized homogenized skim milk. Pasteurization, like antibiotics, kills both good and harmful bacteria. The process also destroys the beneficial enzymes in milk, which makes milk harder to digest. As I said earlier, whole organic milk is very good, goat's milk is even better, and cultured or fermented dairy is the very best.

9. Hydrolyzed soy protein. If you're wondering what in the world this is, hydrolyzed soy protein is another difficult-to-digest substance found in imitation meat products. It's produced by an extraction process of hydrolysis in which soybeans are boiled in a vat of acid and then neutralized with a caustic soda. A sludge forms on the top and is allowed to dry before being scraped off. As part of the hydrolyzation process, this soy-based product produces free glutamic acid, which is similar to the flavor-enhancing monosodium glutamate (MSG), which is a neurotoxic substance.

Stick to the real stuff.

10. Artificial flavors and colors. These are never good for you under the best of circumstances, and certainly not when you're trying to ease digestive pain.

11. Excessive alcohol. Drinking alcohol contributes to heartburn in several ways. Alcohol consumption can increase the relaxation of the lower esophageal sphincter, which is manifested by a good beer burp and a jolt of pain in the esophagus. Too much drinking results in overtime production of stomach acids, and alcohol can make the esophagus more sensitive to harsh acid in its protective lining. If that isn't enough to prompt you to exercise caution with drinking, alcohol is also a leading cause of ulcers, gastritis, and pancreatitis.

Finally, long-term, excessive drinking damages every organ in the body (especially the liver), adds weight, produces heart problems, promotes depression, and impacts fertility. Enough said?

12. Chewing gum. Don't chew on a piece of gum between meals. Slapping a stick of chewing gum in your mouth and chewing away start those valuable digestive juices flowing—but then nothing gets sent down the hatch! Chewing a stick of gum wastes important starch-digesting enzymes found in saliva and creates an environment for heartburn. Since gum is full of sugars, artificial sweeteners, and chemicals anyway, it's best not to chew gum at all.

EAT: What Foods Are Extraordinary, Average, or Trouble?

I've prepared a comprehensive list of foods that are ranked in descending order based on their health-giving qualities. The best foods to serve and eat are what I call "Extraordinary," which God created for us to eat and will give you the best chance not to experience heartburn or acid reflux. If you are battling one of the digestive afflictions, however, it is best to consume foods from the Extraordinary category more than 75 percent of the time.

Foods in the Average category should make up less than 25 percent of your daily diet. If you're in the throes of heartburn and acid reflux pain, consume these foods sparingly.

Foods in the Trouble category should be consumed with extreme caution. If you are dealing with heartburn or acid reflux in any manner, you should avoid these foods completely.

For a complete listing of Extraordinary, Average, and Trouble Foods, visit www.BiblicalHealthInstitute.com/EAT.

Practice Fasting Once a Week

If your stomach does a break dance every time you eat a spicy tamale or your esophagus spasms in pain following a meat-and-potatoes dinner, then I urge you to practice a partial fast once a week. I'm a firm believer in giving the body's midsection time off from the round-the-clock digestive cycle, which could ease abdominal stress and indigestion.

If I had heartburn or acid reflux, my attitude about fasting would be: *What do I have to lose?* You may find that fasting is the pause that refreshes. Taking a sustained break from eating will improve your physical health in ways you can't understand, but there's a spiritual side to fasting that must be addressed as well. Something about denying your growling stomach leads to greater self-control and opens one up, I believe, to hearing what God wants to say to you.

The Bible is full of references to fasting—seventy-four in all—and tells how spiritual giants such as David, Daniel, and Paul experienced periods of fasting before launching themselves into doing God's work. When you fast and pray (two words that seem to go hand in hand in

Scripture), you are pursuing God in your life and opening yourself to experiencing a renewed sense of well-being and dependence upon the Lord.

For those with heartburn, I think it's better—and more realistic—to concentrate on completing a one-day partial fast once a week. In this type of fast, you wake up in the morning and refrain from eating breakfast and lunch, as well as any snacks. Then you resume eating with a dinner-time meal.

If you've never voluntarily fasted for a day, I urge you to try it—and I'm betting your tender esophagus will thank you for the rest.

℞ THE GREAT PHYSICIAN'S RX FOR HEARTBURN AND ACID REFLUX: EAT TO LIVE

- *Eat only foods God created.*

- *Eat foods in a form that is healthy for the body.*

- *Consume foods high in fiber, such as fruits and vegetables.*

- *Consume an apple cider vinegar and honey drink daily.*

- *Consume liberal amounts of homemade chicken soup.*

- *Consume foods high in omega-3 fatty acids like wild-caught fish.*

- *Avoid foods high in sugar.*

- *Avoid foods containing hydrogenated oils.*

- *Lay off alcohol, chocolate, and mints.*

- *Drink plenty of water.*

Take Action

To learn how to incorporate the principles of eating to live into your daily lifestyle, please turn to page 75 for the Great Physician's Rx for Heartburn and Acid Reflux Battle Plan.

KEY #2

Supplement Your Diet with Whole Food Nutritionals, Living Nutrients, and Superfoods

T*um-ta-tum-tum-TUMS* . . .

When a gastric volcano erupts beneath the breastbone, you'll do most anything to shut off the lava flow, like popping something into your mouth to bring about fast, effective relief. That's how millions of Americans cope with digestive distress after digging into an Italian sausage pizza washed down with ample amounts of pale ale.

Antacids, as I mentioned in the introduction, are the first medication that folks like Tim Roos reach for when heartburn pain strikes. Although you can choose from dozens of different brands filling supermarket and pharmacy shelves, nearly all antacids rely on three basic ingredients to get the job done: magnesium, aluminum, and calcium.

Popping antacids like party hors d'oeuvres can introduce too much of a not-so-good thing into the digestive tract, however. A major side effect of too much magnesium is diarrhea. A major side effect of too much aluminum is constipation. And too much calcium can inhibit protein digestion and lead to kidney failure as well as dizziness, nausea, and vomiting.

I think you should take *something* to deal with heartburn and acid reflux, but I don't think ingesting medications or antacids to mask heartburn pain is the best way to go. A better route is taking a few key nutritional supplements *before* the onset of heartburn pain, which will better prepare your gut to receive and process the food that wends its way through the digestive tract.

I believe that sufferers of heartburn and acid reflux must introduce probiotics and digestive enzymes into their bodies as well as green foods, which are also known as "superfoods." The best supplements are capsules and caplets made with raw materials that are known in the industry as "whole food" or "living" nutritional supplements. When it comes to dealing with heartburn and acid reflux, supplementing your diet with whole food nutritionals, living nutrients, and superfoods can go a long way toward helping you unlock your health potential.

Let's begin with probiotics, a term you may not be familiar with. Probiotics are living, direct-fed microbials (DFMs) that promote the growth of beneficial bacteria in the intestines. The lack of probiotics in our diet is a contributing reason why millions are afflicted with intestinal problems like gastritis, ulcerative colitis, and acid reflux. Our society has developed an antibiotic culture so intent on destroying bacteria that we've eradicated much of the beneficial bacteria in our bodies and the environment, thanks to the development of antibiotic drugs, the introduction of chlorinated water, the onset of air pollution, and the continued reliance on a poor diet.

I'll never forget the impact that probiotic supplements with soil-based organisms (SBOs) had on me when I made my health comeback a dozen years ago. Natasha Trenev, author of *Probiotics: Nature's Internal Healers* and a recognized authority on the subject for thirty years, points out that a bacteria named

Lactobacillus bulgaricus has been found to be very effective for alleviating digestive problems like acid reflux. "Beneficial *L. bulgaricus* colonies form a hostile environment for pathogenic or disease-causing germs and play a major detoxification role in removing potentially harmful germs that travel through the G. I. tract," she wrote[1]. Other members of the *Lactobacillus* family are *Lactobacillus acidophilus* and *Lactobacillus casei.*

Soil-based organisms are beneficial organisms found in soil, which exhibit the same health-enhancing characteristics of probiotics supplements. "When taken as a supplement, SBOs help detoxify the intestinal tract, improve nutrient absorption, and expel pathogens, including parasites," say the authors of *Alternative Medicine: The Definitive Guide.* "Research has shown that SBOs facilitate overall cellular health and . . . enhance immune function due to their antioxidant properties."[2]

Dietary supplements that contain these probiotics are a great way to reintroduce helpful microorganisms into your digestive tract, which can improve bowel and immune system function, increase nutrient absorption, and detoxify the body and its organs. I think the best probiotics are the ones that contain multiple strains of microorganisms containing *Lactobacillus, Bacillus,* and *Saccharomyces* species in a base of ionic plant-based minerals. (I know I've become very technical in this description of probiotics, but the reason I know a great deal about these microorganisms is that I studied how they work following my two-year bout with various digestive ailments and diseases that nearly claimed my life.)

Digestive enzymes rank right up there with probiotics because they help prevent heartburn by assisting in the breakdown of difficult-to-digest foods, especially carbohydrates. You need to be aware that digestive enzymes come with various ratios of different enzymes. For instance, as a chronic heartburn sufferer, you may want to avoid digestive enzymes that contain large amounts of proteases, which break down protein. Too much protease has been reported to aggravate ulcers and gastritis. I recommend the consumption of a plant-based enzyme product containing large amounts of carbohydrate-digesting enzymes including maltase, lactase, cellulose, and phytase.

Digestive enzymes aid digestion and can help remove sticky waste that adheres to the lining of the intestines. They are the body's day laborers, the ones responsible for synthesizing, delivering, and eliminating the unbelievable number of ingredients and chemicals that your body uses during the waking hours. Normally, our foods contain natural digestive enzymes, but cooking foods above 130 degrees Fahrenheit or eating processed foods (just about everything sold on a shelf in a supermarket) destroys digestive enzymes. Look for comprehensive digestive enzymes products with more than two dozen different digestive enzymes to ensure that your stomach is receiving the digestive enzymes it needs to break down foods into nutrients that the body can readily assimilate.

Next on my list is a green food supplement that's a blend of barley, wheat, oat, and alfalfa grass juices combined with other vegetables, tart fruits, microalgae such as spirulina and chlorella, and sprouted grains and seeds. Green foods, or superfoods, are high in minerals, enzymes, and chlorophyll, as you would expect for grasses. Green foods are also alkalizing, which helps to balance stomach acid.

Since so few Americans consume the recommended five servings of vegetables per day—it's generally considered to be less than 10 percent—those who aren't getting their veggies are depriving themselves of nutrient-rich foods that could ward off heartburn and acid reflux. You can add green food powder to liquid or take it in caplet form. Go to www.BiblicalHealthInsitute.com and click on the Resource Guide for recommendations.

Alkalizing Wonders

Macit Gurol, a scientific generalist and holder of numerous US patents, often experienced a severe case of heartburn when he drank his morning coffee. He set forth to formulate a food additive to control acids in foods and beverages, and by golly, he came up with something. Mr. Gurol called his formula AlkaPlex.

AlkaPlex is a proprietary combination of dietary minerals designed to maintain healthy pH levels by providing a mild alkalizing effect. The granules are made by using calcium carbonate powder mined from a pure source in Tennessee, which becomes a carrier for magnesium hydroxide, potassium hydroxide, and potassium chloride. These carrier particles are formed, or agglomerated, into granules using their patented process to maintain a controlled release rate of the ingredients in the gut.

AlkaPlex and other supplements containing alkalizing minerals from goat's milk whey and carrot, beet, and barley juice are well worth checking out if you're dealing with painful heartburn and acid reflux. Goat's milk whey is soothing and healing to the digestive tract because it's the most like human milk in composition. As mentioned in the previous chapter, the composition and size of goat's milk fat globules are five to ten times smaller than those found in the milk of cows.

Since production of highly acidic gastric juice is a normal function of the stomach, it makes sense to take a supplement that contains alkalizing minerals made of goat's milk whey as well as barley grass and beet and carrot juice concentrates.

Finally, I recommend that you round out your nutritional program by taking living multivitamins in whole food form, which are vitamins and minerals that have been fermented with probiotic microorganisms and their enzymes. These also contain a broad array of antioxidants from fruits, vegetables, herbs, and spices. Everyone, especially someone with heartburn problems, needs to take a living multivitamin. A probiotic with SBOs and living multivitamins are a fantastic one-two punch—not *to* your stomach but *for* your stomach.

Remember, you'll find a list of such products at www.Biblical HealthInstitute.com by clicking on the Resource Guide.

R̶x THE GREAT PHYSICIAN'S RX FOR HEARTBURN AND ACID REFLUX: SUPPLEMENT YOUR DIET WITH WHOLE FOOD NUTRITIONALS, LIVING NUTRIENTS, AND SUPERFOODS

- *Probiotics are available in two formats: food and dietary supplements. Be sure to introduce these beneficial microorganisms to your diet daily.*

- *Take digestive enzymes and a whole food living multivitamin with each meal.*

- *Take a green food blend twice per day, morning and evening.*

- *Supplement with AlkaPlex alkalizing mineral complex to reduce acid and enhance alkalinity.*

Take Action

To learn how to incorporate the principles of supplementing your diet with whole food nutritionals, living nutrients, and superfoods, please turn to page 75 for the Great Physician's Rx for Heartburn and Acid Reflux Battle Plan.

KEY #3

Practice Advanced Hygiene

In the last chapter, I talked about how heartburn and acid reflux sufferers should introduce into their bodies probiotics, which are beneficial bacteria that the stomach and digestive tract utilize to keep things on an even keel.

You're probably unaware of this, but every day of your life, your body wards off gazillions of germs that seek to break down your immune system and make you more susceptible to health problems. The idea behind the practice of advanced hygiene, which is the third key that will unlock your health potential, is that protecting your body from viruses and other bugs that can wreak havoc on your digestive system is something you want to do. When you can reduce the number of biological irritants and toxins trying to gain a foothold inside your body, you will be placing less stress on your immune system.

Like breathing and blinking, your body's immune system reacts automatically to any invasion of infection. When you touch a contaminated surface or shake hands or touch someone else, you risk being invaded by disease-causing bacteria, fungi, viruses, and allergens. That leaves you susceptible to developing a digestive problem, especially an ulcer, which researchers believe may be caused by bacterial overgrowth.

Proper hygiene, which is defined as keeping the body clean of toxins, pollutants, and disease-causing germs, is an essential part of the Great Physician's Rx for heartburn and acid reflux. Practicing an advanced hygiene program lightens the load on the immune system and rids your body of germs just itching to get inside your digestive system and create even more mayhem.

I've been practicing an advanced hygiene protocol for more than a decade and witnessed astonishing results in my life: no lingering head colds, no nagging sinus infections, no acute respiratory illnesses to speak of, as well as no heartburn or acid reflux. When I do pick up a bug—and it seems that always happens after a long plane flight—my illnesses are short-lived thanks to an advanced hygiene program first developed by an Australian scientist, Kenneth Seaton, Ph.D. This pioneering researcher discovered that ear, nose, throat, and skin problems can be linked to the fact that humans touch their noses, eyes, and mouths with germ-carrying fingernails throughout the day.

In scientific terms, this is known as auto- or self-inoculation. So how do your fingernails get dirty? Through hand-to-hand contact with surfaces and other people. If you thought that most germs were spread by airborne exposure—someone sneezing at your table—you would be wrong. "Germs don't fly, they hitchhike," Dr. Seaton declared, and he's right.

Dr. Seaton estimates that once you pick up hitchhiking germs, they hibernate and hide around the fingernails, no matter how short you keep them trimmed. You would be surprised to find out how much you scratch your nose or rub your mouth and eyes. If you're like most people, it's a constant habit. When you come into contact with contagious germs, you can get sick, come down with the common cold, or find yourself battling the flu. This happens all the time. Chuck Gerba, a University of Arizona environmental microbiology professor, says that 80 percent of infections, from cold and flu viruses to food-borne diseases, are spread through contact with hands and surfaces.

How do you get germs on your hands? By shaking hands with others or touching things they touched: handrails, doorknobs, shopping carts, paper money, coins, and food. I know this stuff isn't pleasant conversation, but practicing advanced hygiene has become an everyday habit for me. Since I'm aware that 90 percent of germs take up residence around my fingernails, I use a creamy semisoft soap rich in essential oils. Each morning and evening, I dip both of my hands into the tub of semisoft soap and dig my fingernails into the cream. Then I work the special cream around the tips of fingers, cuticles, and fingernails for fifteen to thirty seconds. When I'm finished, I lather my hands for fifteen seconds before rinsing them under running water. After my hands are clean, I take another dab of semisoft soap and wash my face.

My next step involves a procedure that I call a "facial dip." I fill my washbasin or a clean large bowl with warm but not hot water. When enough water is in the basin, I add one to two tablespoons of regular table salt and two eyedroppers of a mineral-based facial solution into the cloudy water. I mix everything with my hands, and then I bend over and dip my face into the cleansing matter, opening my eyes several times to allow the membranes to be cleansed. After coming up for air, I dunk my head a second time and blow bubbles through my nose. "Sink snorkeling," I call it.

My final steps of advanced hygiene involve the application of very dilute drops of hydrogen peroxide and minerals into my ears for thirty to sixty seconds to cleanse the ear canal, followed by brushing my teeth with an essential oil tooth solution to cleanse my teeth, gums, and mouth of unhealthy germs. (For more information on my favorite advanced hygiene products, visit www.BiblicalHealthInstitute.com and click on the Resource Guide.)

Brushing your teeth well and regularly practicing advanced hygiene require discipline; you have to remind yourself to do it until it becomes an ingrained habit. I find it easier to follow these steps in the morning when I'm freshly awake than later in the evening when I'm tired and bleary eyed—although I do my best to practice advanced hygiene mornings and evenings and hardly ever miss.

Either way, it only takes three minutes or so to complete all of the advanced hygiene steps. When it comes to prevention, practicing advanced hygiene three minutes a day makes sense for your tender stomach and digestive system.

A Primer on Washing Your Hands

1. Wet your hands with warm water. It doesn't have to be anywhere near scalding hot.

2. Apply plenty of soap to the palms of both hands. The best soap to use is a semisoft soap that you can dig your fingernails into.

3. Rub your hands vigorously together and scrub all the surfaces. Pay attention to the skin between the fingers and work the soap into the fingernails.

4. Rub and scrub for fifteen to thirty seconds, or about the time it takes to slowly sing "Happy Birthday."

5. Rinse well and dry your hands on a paper towel or clean cloth towel. If you're in a public restroom, it's a good idea to turn off the running water with the towel in your hand. An even *better* idea is to use that same towel to open the door since that door handle is the first place that non-washers touch after they've gone to the bathroom.

6. Keep waterless sanitizers in your purse or wallet, in case soap and water are not available in the public restroom. These towelettes, although not ideal, are better than nothing.

When to Wash Your Hands

- After you go to the bathroom
- Before and after you insert and remove contact lenses
- Before and after food preparation
- Before you eat

- After you sneeze, cough, or blow your nose

- After cleaning up after your pet

- After handling money

- After changing a diaper

- After blowing a child's nose

- After handling garbage

- After cleaning your toilets

- After shaking a bunch of hands

- After shopping at the supermarket

- After attending an event at a public theater

- Before and after sexual intercourse

℞ THE GREAT PHYSICIAN'S RX FOR HEARTBURN AND ACID REFLUX: PRACTICE ADVANCED HYGIENE

- *Dig your fingers into a semisoft soap with essential oils, and wash your hands regularly, paying special attention to removing germs from underneath your fingernails.*

- *Cleanse your nasal passageways and the mucous membranes of the eyes daily by performing a facial dip.*

- *Cleanse the ear canals at least twice per week.*

- *Use an essential oil-based tooth solution daily to remove germs from the teeth, gums, and mouth.*

Take Action

To learn how to incorporate the principles of practicing advanced hygiene, please turn to page 75 for the Great Physician's Rx for Heartburn and Acid Reflux Battle Plan.

KEY #4

Condition Your Body with Exercise and Body Therapies

You could say that when it comes to heartburn, exercise gives new meaning to the term *feeling the burn*.

Everyone agrees that exercise is good for the body, but heartburn sufferers are painfully aware that working out can also induce episodes of heartburn and acid reflux. Vigorous physical effort that requires you to bounce up and down—I'm thinking about jogging, step aerobics, and jumping rope—jostles the sensitive stomach, causing acidic juices to slosh around and sneak through the lower esophageal sphincter into the esophagus. Those brave enough—or dumb enough—to perform sit-ups experience a two-fer: not only do sit-ups force you to clench the abdominal muscles surrounding your stomach, but lying on your back takes away the normal gravitational flow of food into your stomach. Potentially irritating stomach acids have an easier time careening into hypersensitive esophageal tissue when you're lying flat on your back.

That's why many dealing with chronic heartburn and acid reflux find it easier to pack it in and veg out around the house instead of packing up a duffel bag and heading to the gym. According to a study commissioned by the makers of Pepcid, 40 percent of weekly heartburn sufferers have stopped being physically active as a result of their heartburn. Those who do work out say they experience heartburn 45 percent of the time while they exercise. "In a sense, it's a double-whammy," said Steven Peikin, M.D., professor of medicine at Robert Woods Johnson Hospital and author of *Gastrointestinal Health.* "People try to be more healthy by exercising more, but end up inducing heartburn and acid reflux, which not only causes discomfort but also takes them off the road to better overall health."[1]

I know a smoother way to better health, and it's called *functional fitness,* a form of mild exercise that gently works your tender abdominal region, raises your heartbeat, strengthens the body's core muscles, and gives you an emotional lift at a time when life isn't so red hot.

The idea behind functional fitness is to train movements, not muscles, through performing real-life activities in real-life positions. Functional fitness can be done with no equipment or by employing dumbbells, stability balls, or even canned vegetables from your pantry. Here's an example: weighted reaching lunges can be accomplished with a can of tomato sauce, a water bottle, or a light dumbbell. With both hands at your sides holding a weight, step forward with one leg while keeping the other leg as straight as possible. Reach forward with your arms as far as possible.

Do this ten times. Then you can rest your arms at your sides and raise one arm toward the ceiling or sky. (For more information on functional fitness videos and movements, visit www.BiblicalHealthInstitute.com.)

If you feel up to exercising outside your home, then check out functional fitness classes at gyms around the country, including LA Fitness, Bally Total Fitness, and local YMCAs. You'll be asked to perform squats with feet apart, feet together, and one back with the other forward. You'll be asked to do reaching lunges, push-ups against a wall, and "supermans" that involve lying on the floor and lifting up your right arm while lifting your left leg into a fully extended position. What you *won't* be asked to perform are high-impact exercises like those found in pulsating aerobics classes, or what I call "Heartburn Alley."

I have a background in physical fitness, having been a certified fitness trainer. If you were my client, who had been told by the doctor that you have a severe case of acid reflux, I would urge you to start a functional fitness program. This gentle exercise stimulates intestinal activity that keeps the bowels moving, which is just the ticket for those with indigestion troubles or constipation. Some functional fitness programs employ a mini trampoline or rebounder, which, if done correctly, can be performed without jarring jumping. By grabbing a stabilizing bar and gently bouncing up and down, you can increase lymphatic flow while being kind to the digestive tract.

If functional fitness isn't your cup of tea, then try walking. This low-impact exercise places a gentle strain on the hips and the rest of the body, and when done briskly, it makes the heart work harder and expend more energy. Best of all, you can walk when it fits your schedule—before work, on your lunch hour, before dinner, or after dinner. You set the pace; you decide how much you put into this exercise. Walking is a great social exercise that allows you to carry on a civilized conversation with a friend or loved one. Or if you prefer, you can walk on a treadmill at home or at a fitness center. A home treadmill also makes sense in a frigid climate or an area where you feel unsafe walking after dark.

You need to be intentional about incorporating other body therapies into your lifestyle. For instance, let's talk about sleep, which is no lullaby for many heartburn sufferers. As many as one in four Americans suffers from nighttime heartburn, according to a recent study published in the medical journal *Chest*. The figure is even higher among those who have chronic indigestion.[2]

Since lying flat aggravates heartburn symptoms, raising the head of your bed four to six inches (by placing blocks underneath the headboard) elevates your head and chest, which alleviates pressure on the lower esophageal sphincter. Heartburn sufferers can help out by eating dinner at least two to three hours prior to retiring.

How many hours of sleep are you getting nightly? The magic number is eight hours, say the sleep experts. That's because when people are allowed to sleep as much as they would like in a controlled setting, like in a sleep laboratory, they naturally sleep eight hours in a twenty-four-hour time period.

LET THE SUN SHINE IN

You may not see much correlation between sunning yourself and heartburn, but let me explain. When your face or your arms and legs are exposed to sunlight, your skin synthesizes vitamin D from the ultraviolet rays of sunlight. The body needs vitamin D, which is not a vitamin but actually a critical hormone that helps regulate the health of more than thirty tissues and organs, including the digestive tract. I recommend intentionally exposing yourself to at least fifteen minutes of sunlight a day—preferably before 10:00 a.m. or after 2:00 p.m. to avoid the sun's strongest rays—to increase vitamin D levels in the body.

But if you really want to pamper yourself, try hydrotherapy. Sitting in a sauna or taking a steam bath is a form of hydrotherapy that is beneficial because of the way it causes accumulated toxins and impactions to release. A great way to detoxify the body of harmful environmental chemicals, fat-soluble toxins, and heavy metals is the regular use of a far infrared sauna. Far infrared saunas gently raise the heart rate and improve metabolism. I have owned and used a far infrared sauna for more than eight years and highly recommend it. (For more information on far infrared sauna technology, visit www.BiblicalHealthInstitute.com.)

Hydrotherapy also comes in the form of baths, showers, washing, and wraps—using hot *and* cold water. For instance, I wake up with a hot shower in the morning, but then I turn off the hot water and stand under the brisk cold water for about a minute, which totally invigorates me. Cold water stimulates the body and boosts oxygen use in the cells, while hot water dilates blood vessels, which improves blood circulation and transports more oxygen to the brain. I can remember when I had major cramps around the abdomen and let a stream of hot and then cold water hit the abdominal area. I always felt better after this water massage.

Finally, pamper yourself with aromatherapy and music therapy. In aromatherapy, essential oils from plants, flowers, and spices are introduced to your skin and pores either by rubbing them in or by inhaling their aromas. The use of these essential oils can give you an emotional lift. Try rubbing a few drops of myrtle, coriander, hyssop, galbanum, or frankincense onto the palms, then cup your hands over your mouth and nose and inhale. A deep breath will invigorate the spirit.

So will listening to soft and soothing music that promotes relaxation and healing. I know what I like when it comes to music therapy: contemporary praise and worship music. No matter what works for you, you'll find that listening to uplifting mood music can heal the body, soul, and spirit.

Rx THE GREAT PHYSICIAN'S RX FOR HEARTBURN AND ACID REFLUX: CONDITION YOUR BODY WITH EXERCISE AND BODY THERAPIES

- *Make a commitment to exercise three times a week or more.*

- *Incorporate five to fifteen minutes of functional fitness into your daily schedule.*

- *Take a brisk walk and see how much better you feel at the end of the day.*

- *Make a conscious effort to practice deep-breathing exercises once a day. Inflate your lungs to full and hold for several seconds before slowly exhaling.*

- *Go to sleep earlier, paying close attention to how much sleep you get before midnight. Do your best to get eight hours of sleep nightly. Remember that sleep is the most important nonnutrient you can incorporate into your health regimen.*

- *End your shower by changing the water temperature to cool (or cold) and standing underneath the spray for one minute.*

- *Each Saturday or Sunday, take a day of rest. Dedicate the day to the Lord and do something fun and relaxing that you haven't done in a while. Make your rest day work-free, errand-free, and shop-free. Trust God that He'll do more with His six days than you can do with seven.*

- *Once each day, sit outside in a chair and face the sun. Soak up the rays for ten or fifteen minutes.*

- *Incorporate essential oils into your daily life.*

- *Play worship music in your home, in your car, or on your iPod. Focus on God's plan for your life.*

Take Action

To learn how to incorporate the principles of conditioning
your body with exercise and body therapies into your
daily lifestyle, please turn to page 75 for the Great
Physician's Rx for Heartburn and Acid Reflux Battle Plan.

KEY #5

Reduce Toxins in Your Environment

I like what the cheeky Web site wrongdiagnosis.com had to say about heartburn: "Certain medications, chemicals, toxins, or substances may possibly be underlying causes of heartburn. Side effects of medications, or exposure to toxins, chemicals, or other substances may cause a symptom or condition. Hence, they become possible underlying causes of heartburn but are often misdiagnosed or overlooked as a cause."[1]

If you're dealing with chronic heartburn, acid reflux, or GERD, there's a good chance you have an imbalanced body trying to deal with an overload of environmental and bacterial toxins in your digestive tract. Elaine Gottschall, author of *Breaking the Vicious Cycle,* explained it this way: "Although there is still insufficient evidence to link a specific microbe to each of the chronic intestinal disorders, it is generally agreed that intestinal microbes are not innocent bystanders."[2]

It would be naive not to believe that some mean toxins are out there, just waiting for their chance to invade your gut. What kinds of toxins are we talking about?

In a study led by the Mount Sinai School of Medicine in New York, in collaboration with the Environmental Working Group and Commonweal, researchers at two major laboratories found an average of ninety-one industrial compounds, pollutants, and other chemicals in the blood and urine of nine volunteers. A partial listing of the contaminants found in the volunteer test group revealed that many had traces of toxins such as PCBs (polychlorinated biphenyls), dioxins, furans, metals, asbestos, organochlorine insecticides (the long name for pesticides such as DDT and chlordane), phthalates, VOCs (volatile organic compounds), and chlorine.[3]

The nine volunteers in the Mount Sinai study did not work with chemicals on the job or live downwind from polluting smokestacks when they were scanned for 210 toxic substances. Of the 167 chemicals found in their blood and urine, 76 cause cancer in humans or animals, 94 are toxic to the brain and nervous system, and 79 cause birth defects or abnormal development in children. Scientists refer to this chemical residue as a person's body burden.

Although our bodies are designed to eliminate toxins, our immune systems have become overloaded to the point that they're on perpetual tilt! What happens is that our bodies can absorb and excrete water-soluble chemical toxins just fine, but fat-soluble chemicals such as dioxins, phthalates, and chlorine are stored in our fatty tissues, where it takes months or even years for these toxins to be eliminated from our systems. This can put a massive strain on your digestive tract.

That's why the Great Physician's prescription for heartburn and acid reflux calls for eating leaner meat since fats in conventional or nonorganic meats act as chemical magnets for toxins in the environment. Certain types of fish and shellfish should be avoided to lower your exposure to mercury. Choosing organic produce will lower the level of pesticides in your body. You should thoroughly wash your fruits and veggies no matter where you do your shopping—a supermarket, health food store, or farmer's roadside stand.

Up in the Air

Harmful toxins are in the air as well. Today's well-insulated homes and energy-efficient windows and doors trap "used" air with harmful particles of carbon dioxide, nitrogen dioxide, and pet dander. When the US Environmental Protection Agency (EPA) conducted a survey of six hundred homes in six cities, researchers discovered that peak concentrations of twenty toxic compounds were hundreds of times higher *inside* homes than outside. "If we measured outdoors what we are measuring indoors," said EPA spokesperson Lance Wallace, "there would be a tremendous cry to clean up outdoor air."[4]

Opening your doors and windows to let fresh air flow into your home should be done several times a day, no matter what the temperature is like outside. Even in Florida's sticky summer heat, my wife, Nicki, and I will periodically air out the house, and sometimes we'll sleep with a window cracked open in the master bedroom. We've also set up four air purifiers inside our home, which clean room air through electrical charges to capture airborne particles, microbes, and molds. Air purifiers are a wonderful technology that's becoming more affordable each year.

Carcinogenic contaminants are found in a variety of popular household products, including cleaners and cosmetics. Regarding the former, the less contact with chemical-rich kitchen cleansers, oven cleaner, glues, paints, paint thinner, and other solvents the better.

The idea is to use natural ingredients such as vinegar, lemon juice, baking soda, and commercially available natural cleansers to clean your home to a spick-and-span and high-sheen gloss. A solution of one cup vinegar in a pail of water is all you need to mop the kitchen floor, make kitchen sinks shine, and sanitize toilets. *The Safe Shopper's Bible* is a superb resource for offering alternatives to toxin-producing products such as:

- air fresheners
- all-purpose cleaners
- bathroom cleaners and disinfectants
- bleaches
- carpet cleaners
- deodorizers
- scouring powders
- soft scrubs
- toilet bowl deodorizers
- dishwashing detergents
- drain openers
- floor cleaners
- floor waxes
- oven cleaners
- furniture polishes

- upholstery cleaners

- silver polish

- glass and window cleaners

- laundry detergents

- fabric softeners

- stain removers

- laundry starches

That's quite a list, but I bet you didn't know that you had so many potentially toxic household cleaners under your kitchen sink, in your laundry room, or in your garage. Cleaning products, wood and silver polishes, cans of paint, and liquid solvents don't belong inside the house. Store them in the garage or, preferably, in a backyard storage shed.

Better yet, search out natural substitutes in *The Safe Shopper's Bible*. Lemon juice will shine up brass and copper, and when mixed with olive oil, it works fine as a furniture polish. Baking soda takes on the dirty chore of scrubbing toilets, sinks, and showers as well as Mr. Clean.

Last, I must point out the toxic qualities of cosmetics, hair dyes, and hairsprays in your bathroom cabinets. Eye shadow, mascara, makeup, and lipstick are put directly on the skin. We know how absorbent skin is since your skin absorbs chlorine when you take a shower, and if you rub crushed garlic cloves on your feet, you may have garlic breath in twenty minutes. You can find natural cosmetics in progressive groceries and natural food stores nationwide, or visit www.BiblicalHealthInstitute.com and click on the Resource Guide for recommended products.

Let me leave you with this thought regarding toxins in your environment. As a defense, some scientists will quote Paracelsus, the famous medieval alchemist who said hundreds of years ago, "It's the dose that makes the poison." In other words, if the toxic dose is low enough, the body can handle it.

To me, it's not a coincidence that toxins in the environment are climbing just as the ranks of those with heartburn and acid reflux are increasing each year. That's why we must be proactive in reducing toxins in our personal environments.

℞ THE GREAT PHYSICIAN'S RX FOR HEARTBURN AND ACID REFLUX: REDUCE TOXINS IN YOUR ENVIRONMENT

- *Consume organically produced food as much as possible.*

- *Improve indoor air quality by opening windows, changing air filters regularly, setting out house-plants, and buying an air filtration system.*

- *Drink only purified water.*

- *Shower in purified water.*

- *Use natural products for skin care, body care, hair care, and cosmetics.*

- *Don't heat food in plastic.*

- *Don't cook with microwave ovens.*

- *Don't cook with nonstick cookware.*

- *Don't smoke cigarettes or use tobacco products.*

- *Use natural cleaning products for your home, washing machine, and dishwasher.*

Take Action

To learn how to incorporate the principles of reducing toxins in your environment into your daily lifestyle, please turn to page 75 for the Great Physician's Rx for Heartburn and Acid Reflux Battle Plan.

KEY #6

Avoid Deadly Emotions

Tell me I've seen this made-for-TV movie somewhere before.

The scene: a well-appointed corner office in a New York City skyscraper overlooking Central Park. The camera focuses on the tension-riddled face of the dressed-for-success female CEO, who's on the phone juggling the fortunes of a billion-dollar company and the lives of thousands of employees with the demands of a husband and two elementary school kids who need her.

When she has a free moment, she pensively reaches into her compact for a couple of antacids to take the edge off. That's what Hollywood screenwriters do when they need to show the protagonist dealing with tons of stress.

Heart-pounding stress is a surefire route to heartburn and a key source for a variety of other ills: hypertension, elevated heartbeat, headaches, and hormonal imbalances in the body. Tension caused by work-related or family-related stress compounds physical problems. What's becoming more and more apparent to researchers is that emotions such as stress, anger, acrimony, apprehension, agitation, anxiety, and alarm are powerful forces within the human mind that clearly affect the body and the soul.

My friend Don Colbert, M.D., author of the fine book *Deadly Emotions,* says that unmediated chronic stress has been linked to a long list of physical problems including heartburn, indigestion, gastritis, ulcers, constipation, and gastroesophageal reflux disease (GERD). Traveling through life on an emotional roller coaster saps a person of both physical and psychological health, which often leaves body and mind depleted of energy and strength. Dr. Colbert points out that medical studies dealing with unhealthy emotions show that the mind and the body are linked, which means how you feel emotionally can determine how you feel physically.

What about you? Are you harboring resentment in your heart, nursing a grudge into overtime, or plotting revenge against those who hurt you? If you're bottling up emotions such as anger, bitterness, and resentment, these deadly emotions will produce toxins similar to bingeing on nachos and jalapenos. The efficiency of your immune system decreases noticeably for six hours, and staying angry and bitter can alter the chemistry of your body. An old proverb states it well: "What you are eating is not nearly as important as what's eating you."

This is the time to put your past in the rearview mirror and move forward. There may be someone in your past that you need to forgive. I learned this lesson when I shared a meal with Bruce Wilkinson, author of *The Prayer of Jabez* and the founder of Walk Thru the Bible Ministries. Over breakfast, he urged me to forgive those who had hurt me in the past by writing his or her name on a piece of paper and then stating, "I forgive you for . . ."

I balked at first, telling Dr. Wilkinson that I wasn't the type to hold grudges. But he persisted, asking me again, "Jordan, is there anyone in your life that you need to forgive?"

Actually there were a couple of doctors who told me that my illnesses were my fault. Several relatives and friends said they would be there for me when I got sick, but I never heard from them again. Bruce Wilkinson was right: there were more people than I would have thought. After I dealt with each person, I bowed my head and asked God to help me forgive these people just as He forgives me for my sins. I prayed with a contrite heart, seeking His mercy and forgiveness.

As for you, please remember that no matter how bad you've been hurt in the past, it's still possible to forgive. Jesus said, "For if you forgive men their trespasses, your heavenly Father will also forgive you. But if you don't forgive men their trespasses, neither will your Father forgive your trespasses" (Matt. 6:14–15 NKJV).

If you're angry, hurt, or bothered by those who've done horrible things to you, give them your forgiveness, and then let it go.

℞ THE GREAT PHYSICIAN'S RX FOR HEARTBURN AND ACID REFLUX: AVOID DEADLY EMOTIONS

- *Recognize the interaction between heartburn and acid reflux and deadly emotions.*

- *Trust God when you face circumstances that cause you to worry or become anxious.*

- *Practice forgiveness every day and forgive those who hurt you.*

Take Action

To learn how to incorporate the principles of avoiding deadly emotions into your daily lifestyle, please turn to page 75 for the Great Physician's Rx for Heartburn and Acid Reflux Battle Plan.

KEY #7

Live of Life of Prayer and Purpose

No matter how much he willed his body to do otherwise, Doug McLean couldn't eat a meal without burping up stinging stomach acid. His heartburn was as regular as Big Ben: within an hour of finishing a meal, the *gong* sounded the start of his chronic acid reflux condition, regardless of what he ate.

"My eating habits became increasingly erratic as this painful condition began to wreak havoc on me emotionally, physically, and socially," he said. "I often ate in seclusion to avoid any embarrassment associated with my condition, which was later determined to be GERD—gastroesophageal reflux disease."

Doug sought medical help, and over an eighteen-month period, he visited every gastrointestinal specialist who was part of his HMO health insurance plan. They ran the usual battery of tests:

- an upper GI series, in which Doug was asked to drink a liquid contrast to coat the esophagus and stomach; X-rays were taken to evaluate the size and shape of the esophagus and detect the presence of a hiatal hernia

- an upper GI endoscopy, in which Doug was given a sedative so that a lighted, flexible tube called an endoscopy with a video camera on the end could be

passed into the esophagus and stomach to inspect the
lining visually

- an esophageal manometry, in which a specialized tube
was passed into the esophagus to measure esophageal
muscle function and the function of the lower
esophageal sphincter

After these invasive tests, you can understand why Doug felt
like running for the hills in his hospital smock every time a doctor approached him to insert a black tube down his throat. When
the tests results came in, however, the verdict was definitive: Doug
had a severe case of GERD complicated by a gaping hiatal hernia,
a duodenal ulcer, and an abnormally slow-emptying stomach,
which emptied 75 percent slower than males his age.

That wasn't the last of the bad news. Because of his severe
acid reflux, Doug was a prime candidate to develop esophageal
cancer. What had been a significant irritant to the quality of
his life was rapidly becoming a life-threatening condition.
Doug began a three-year treatment odyssey that led him to try
various prescription drugs that promised relief but came with
quite noticeable side effects: constant nausea, sleeplessness, and
headaches.

Each month, each week, and each passing episode of painful
GERD moved Doug closer toward the "nuclear" option: submit-
ting to an uncommon surgical procedure known as a laparoscopic
Nissen. This grisly surgery meant that doctors would cut off the
upper one-third of his stomach and tie up what was left of his

stomach to the bottom of his esophagus. This radical approach was needed, his surgeon said. *You don't want to deal with cancer.*

With great reluctance, Doug agreed to submit to a laparoscopic Nissen, and he scheduled a pre-op appointment with a hospital in South Florida. Later that same day, Doug told a colleague at work that he had decided to go forward with the surgery. Doug said he didn't know his coworker very well, but his ears perked up when his friend said, "Have you ever heard of Jordan Rubin?"

"No, I haven't," Doug replied.

His coworker proceeded to describe my miraculous health comeback and how that fueled my passion, vision, and purpose in life, which was to help transform the health of God's people, one life at a time. "Perhaps you should talk to Jordan," his friend suggested. "He might be able to help you."

The first thing Doug did was to check out my Web site (www.jordanrubin.com), where he read about my life-and-death battle with Crohn's disease. Fascinated and inspired, Doug felt hope—the hope that his stomach wouldn't be butchered and he could live a life free of painful acid reflux. Doug didn't know how to contact me, though, so he started with the phone number on the Web site. What happened next was nothing short of a God thing.

Answering the phone call was a customer service representative who sounded vaguely familiar to Doug. As they began talking and Doug shared his story, the customer service rep recognized his old friend. He agreed to go to bat for Doug and ask me to meet with him to see if there was some way I could help.

When we met in person, I immediately saw the look of

concern—and fear—etched on Doug's face. I sought to boost his confidence by saying that I believed the Great Physician's prescription could save him from a date with a scalpel-wielding surgeon. Was he interested in giving it a try?

Doug was all over that, and I outlined many of the ideas found in this book, including two of the most important keys: eating foods that God created in a form healthy for the body and supplementing his diet with probiotics, digestive enzymes, and green foods.

Doug remembers the date he started following the Great Physician's prescription, December 16, 2002, because as God is his witness, that was the *last* day he experienced heartburn and acid reflux. Years of praying for a healing had come to fruition.

If you're in the midst of a gastrointestinal battle with scourges like heartburn and acid reflux, I would imagine that you've been driven to your knees in prayer. There's something about this painful affliction—which isn't well understood by modern medicine and has no sure-shot cure—that causes one to plead for healing from the One who "fearfully and wonderfully made" us (Ps. 139:14 NKJV).

Please be reminded that prayer is the most powerful tool you possess. Prayer connects the entire person—mind, body, and spirit—to God. Prayer is how we talk to God. Prayer is not a formality. Prayer is not about religion. Prayer is about a relationship—the hotline to heaven. We can talk to God anytime, anywhere, for any reason. He is always there to listen, and He always has our best interests at heart because we are His children.

Prayer is the foundation of a healthy life. Prayer is two-way communication with our Creator, the God of the universe. There's power in prayer: "The prayer offered in faith will make the sick person well" (James 5:15 NIV).

The seventh key to unlocking your health potential is living a life of prayer and purpose. Prayer will confirm your purpose, and it will give you the perseverance to complete it. Seal all that you do with the power of prayer, and watch your life become more than you ever thought possible.

FINDING YOUR PURPOSE

"You have a lot to live for."

That saying has become a soothing cliché in our culture, but when you unpack that statement, the fact is, you *do* have a lot to live for. God may have created you with an imperfect stomach or a lousy lower esophageal sphincter, but that doesn't mean He doesn't have great things ahead of you or that He has not given you a purpose in life.

When God took me through two years of horrible sickness before restoring my health, I came out of that experience knowing what my purpose was in life: to share God's message of health and hope so that people wouldn't have to go through what I did. Everything else that I do today is icing—made with raw honey, of course—on the cake. I can't wait to get up in the morning, hoping that I have the privilege of communicating life-changing principles of good health with one person, one thousand people, or even millions that day through radio or television.

If you say to yourself, *I'm not sure I have a purpose,* you would be wrong. If there is air in your lungs, you have a purpose; it's ingrained in your being. If you haven't found your purpose yet, search your heart. What makes you feel alive? What are you passionate about? The joys of family? The arts? Teaching others? Your purpose is waiting to be discovered. Pinpoint your passions, and you'll uncover your purpose. Keep in mind that God gives us different desires, different dreams, and different talents for a reason because we are all part of one body. Having a purpose will give you something to live for.

Don't let heartburn, acid reflux, or GERD keep you down. You can bounce back. You can overcome this affliction with God's help. You have a lot more life to live.

I'm cheering for you because I know you can do it. I urge you to follow the Great Physician's prescription today. I've yet to meet anyone who regretted feeling better and becoming healthier, and you won't either.

Start a Small Group

It's difficult to face the ravages of heartburn and acid reflux alone. If you have friends or family members struggling with similar symptoms, ask them to join you in following the Great Physician's prescription. To learn about joining an existing group in your area or leading a small group in your church, please visit www.BiblicalHealthInstitute.com.

Rx THE GREAT PHYSICIAN'S RX FOR HEARTBURN AND ACID REFLUX: LIVE A LIFE OF PRAYER AND PURPOSE

- Pray continually.

- Confess God's promises upon waking and before you retire.

- Find God's purpose for your life and live it.

- Be an agent of change in your life by adopting the seven keys that will unlock your health potential.

- Find someone you know who is suffering from heartburn or acid reflux and begin the Great Physician's Rx for Heartburn and Acid Reflux Battle Plan together.

Take Action

To learn how to incorporate the principles of living a life of prayer and purpose into your daily lifestyle, please turn to page 75 for the Great Physician's Rx for Heartburn and Acid Reflux Battle Plan.

THE GREAT PHYSICIAN'S RX FOR HEARTBURN AND ACID REFLUX BATTLE PLAN

DAY 1

Upon Waking

Prayer: thank God because this is the day that the Lord has made. Rejoice and be glad in it. Thank Him for the breath in your lungs and the life in your body. Ask the Lord to heal your body and use your experience to benefit the lives of others. Read Matthew 6:9–13 aloud.

Purpose: ask the Lord to give you an opportunity to add significance to someone's life today. Watch for that opportunity. Ask God to use you this day for His intended purpose.

Advanced hygiene: for hands and nails, jab fingers into semisoft soap four or five times, and lather hands with soap for fifteen seconds, rubbing soap over cuticles and rinsing under water as warm as you can stand. Take another swab of semisoft soap into your hands and wash your face. Next, fill the basin or sink with water as warm as you can stand, and add one to three tablespoons of table salt and one to three eyedroppers of iodine-based mineral solution. Dunk face into water and open eyes, blinking repeatedly underwater. Keep eyes open underwater for three seconds. After cleaning your eyes, put your face back in the water and close your mouth while blowing bubbles out of your nose. Come up from the water, and immerse your face in the water once again, gently taking water into your nostrils and expelling bubbles. Come up from the water, and blow your nose into facial tissue.

To cleanse the ears, use hydrogen peroxide and mineral-based ear drops, putting two or three drops into each ear and letting stand for sixty seconds. Tilt your head to expel the drops. For the teeth, apply two or three drops of essential oil–based tooth drops to the toothbrush. This can

75

be used to brush your teeth or added to existing toothpaste. After brushing your teeth, brush your tongue for fifteen seconds. (For recommended advanced hygiene products, visit www.BiblicalHealthInstitute.com and click on the Resource Guide.)

Reduce toxins: open your windows for one hour today. Use natural soap and natural skin and body care products (shower gel, body creams, etc.). Use natural facial care products. Use natural toothpaste. Use natural hair care products such as shampoo, conditioner, gel, mousse, and hairspray. (For recommended products, visit www.BiblicalHealth Institute.com and click on the Resource Guide.)

Morning alkalizing drink: mix the following ingredients in twelve ounces of warm purified water: two teaspoons of organic raw apple cider vinegar, one serving of an alkalizing mineral formula with AlkaPlex, and two teaspoons of raw organic honey. (For recommended products, visit www.BiblicalHealthInstitute.com and click on the Resource Guide.)

Body therapy: get twenty minutes of direct sunlight sometime during the day, but be careful between the hours of 10:00 a.m. and 2:00 p.m.

Exercise: perform functional fitness exercises for five to fifteen minutes or spend five to fifteen minutes on a mini trampoline. (Warning: jumping on a mini trampoline may initially make heartburn symptoms worse, but over time, it can be beneficial.) Finish with five to ten minutes of deep-breathing exercises. (One to three rounds of the exercises can be found at www.BiblicalHealthInstitute.com.)

Emotional health: whenever you face a circumstance, such as your health, that causes you to worry, repeat the following: "Lord, I trust You. I cast my cares upon You, and I believe that You're going to take care of [insert your current situation] and make my health and body strong." Confess that throughout the day whenever you think about your health condition.

Breakfast
Make a smoothie in a blender with the following ingredients:

1 cup plain yogurt or kefir (goat's milk or sheep's milk is best)

1 tablespoon organic flaxseed oil

1 tablespoon organic raw honey

1 cup organic fruit (berries, banana, peaches, etc.)

2 tablespoons goat's milk protein powder (for recommended products, visit www.BiblicalHealthInstitute.com and click on the Resource Guide)

dash of vanilla extract (optional)

Supplements: take one capsule of a probiotic/enzyme blend with soil-based organisms, two caplets of a supergreen formula, and two whole food multivitamin caplets. (For recommended products, visit www.Biblical HealthInstitute.com and click on the Resource Guide.)

Lunch

Before eating, drink eight ounces of water.

During lunch, drink eight ounces of water.

large green salad with mixed greens, avocado, carrots, cucumbers, celery, tomatoes, red cabbage, red peppers, red onions, and sprouts with three hard-boiled omega-3 eggs. Caution: if eating certain raw veggies causes a flare-up of heartburn symptoms, make sure to chew very well and eliminate cabbage, peppers, and onions from the salad.

salad dressing: mix extra virgin olive oil, apple cider vinegar or lemon juice, minced fresh garlic, naturally brewed soy sauce, Celtic Sea Salt, herbs, and spices; or, mix one tablespoon of extra virgin olive oil with one tablespoon of a healthy store-bought dressing

one apple with skin

Supplements: take one capsule of a probiotic/enzyme blend with soil-based organisms, two caplets of a supergreen formula, and two whole food multivitamin caplets.

Dinner

(Please note: If you're suffering from heartburn or acid reflux, it is best to finish dinner by 7:30 p.m. or at least three hours before your normal bedtime.)

During dinner, drink eight to sixteen ounces of water.

baked, poached, or grilled wild-caught salmon

steamed broccoli

large green salad with mixed greens, avocado, carrots, cucumbers, celery, tomatoes, red cabbage, red peppers, red onions, and sprouts. Caution: if eating certain raw veggies causes a flare-up of heartburn symptoms, make sure to chew very well and eliminate cabbage, peppers, and onions from the salad.

salad dressing: mix extra virgin olive oil, apple cider vinegar or lemon juice, minced fresh garlic, naturally brewed soy sauce, Celtic Sea Salt, herbs, and spices; or, mix one tablespoon of extra virgin olive oil with one tablespoon of a healthy store-bought dressing

Supplements: take one capsule of a probiotic/enzyme blend with soil-based organisms, two caplets of a supergreen formula, and two whole food multivitamin caplets.

Snacks

apple slices with raw almond butter

whole food nutrition bar with beta-glucans from soluble oat fiber (for recommended products, visit www.BiblicalHealthInstitute.com and click on the Resource Guide)

eight to twelve ounces of water

Before Bed

Exercise: go for a walk outdoors or participate in a favorite sport or recreational activity.

Evening alkalizing drink: mix the following ingredients in twelve ounces of warm purified water: two teaspoons of organic raw apple cider vinegar, one serving of an alkalizing mineral formula with AlkaPlex, and two teaspoons of raw organic honey. (For recommended products, visit www.BiblicalHealthInstitute.com and click on the Resource Guide.)

Body therapy: take a warm bath for fifteen minutes with eight drops of biblical essential oils added.

Advanced hygiene: repeat the advanced hygiene instructions from the morning of Day 1.

Emotional health: ask the Lord to bring to your mind someone you need to forgive. Take a sheet of paper and write the person's name at the top. Try to remember each specific action that person did against you that brought you pain. Write the following: "I forgive [insert person's name] for [insert the action he or she did against you]." After you fill up the paper, tear it up or burn it, and ask God to give you the strength to truly forgive that person.

Purpose: ask yourself these questions: "Did I live a life of purpose today?" "What did I do to add value to someone else's life today?" Commit to living a day of purpose tomorrow.

Prayer: thank God for this day, asking Him to give you a restoring night's rest and a fresh start tomorrow. Thank Him for His steadfast love that never ceases and His mercies that are new every morning. Read Romans 8:35, 37–39 aloud.

Sleep: go to bed by 10:30 p.m.

Day 2

Upon Waking

Prayer: thank God because this is the day that the Lord has made. Rejoice and be glad in it. Thank Him for the breath in your lungs and the life in your body. Ask the Lord to heal your body and use your experience to benefit the lives of others. Read Psalm 91 aloud.

Purpose: ask the Lord to give you an opportunity to add significance to someone's life today. Watch for that opportunity. Ask God to use you this day for His intended purpose.

Advanced hygiene: follow the advanced hygiene recommendations from the morning of Day 1.

Reduce toxins: follow the recommendations to reduce toxins from the morning of Day 1.

Morning alkalizing drink: mix the following ingredients in twelve ounces of warm purified water: two teaspoons of organic raw apple cider vinegar, one serving of an alkalizing mineral formula with AlkaPlex, and two teaspoons of raw organic honey.

Body therapy: take a hot and cold shower. After a normal shower, alternate sixty seconds of water as hot as you can stand it, followed by sixty seconds of water as cold as you can stand it. Repeat cycle four times for a total of eight minutes, finishing with cold.

Exercise: perform functional fitness exercises for five to fifteen minutes or spend five to fifteen minutes on a mini trampoline. Finish with five to ten minutes of deep-breathing exercises. (One to three rounds of the exercises can be found at www.BiblicalHealthInstitute.com.)

Emotional health: follow the emotional health recommendations from the morning of Day 1.

Breakfast

two or three eggs any style, cooked in one tablespoon of extra virgin coconut oil (for recommended products, visit www.Biblical HealthInstitute.com and click on the Resource Guide)

stir-fried onions, mushrooms, and peppers

one slice of sprouted or yeast-free whole grain bread with almond butter and honey

Supplements: take one capsule of a probiotic/enzyme blend with soil-based organisms, two caplets of a supergreen formula, and two whole food multivitamin caplets.

Lunch

During lunch, drink eight to sixteen ounces of water.

large green salad with mixed greens, avocado, carrots, cucumbers, celery, tomatoes, red cabbage, red peppers, red onions, and sprouts with two ounces of low mercury, high omega-3 tuna (for recommended products, visit www.BiblicalHealthInstitute.com and click on the Resource Guide). Caution: if eating certain raw veggies causes a flare-up of heartburn symptoms, make sure to chew very well and eliminate cabbage, peppers, and onions from the salad.

salad dressing: mix extra virgin olive oil, apple cider vinegar or lemon juice, minced fresh garlic, naturally brewed soy sauce, Celtic Sea Salt, herbs, and spices; or, mix one tablespoon of extra virgin olive oil with one tablespoon of a healthy store-bought dressing

organic grapes

Supplements: take one capsule of a probiotic/enzyme blend with soil-based organisms, two caplets of a supergreen formula, and two whole food multivitamin caplets.

Dinner

(Please note: If you're suffering from heartburn or acid reflux, it is best to finish dinner by 7:30 p.m. or at least three hours before your normal bedtime.)

During dinner, drink eight to sixteen ounces of water.

roasted organic chicken

cooked vegetables (carrots, onions, peas, etc.)

large green salad with mixed greens, avocado, carrots, cucumbers, celery, tomatoes, red cabbage, red peppers, red onions, and sprouts. Caution: if eating certain raw veggies causes a flare-up of heartburn symptoms, make sure to chew very well and eliminate cabbage, peppers, and onions from the salad.

salad dressing: mix extra virgin olive oil, apple cider vinegar or lemon juice, minced fresh garlic, naturally brewed soy sauce, Celtic Sea Salt, herbs, and spices; or, mix one tablespoon of extra virgin olive oil with one tablespoon of a healthy store-bought dressing

Supplements: take one capsule of a probiotic/enzyme blend with soil-based organisms, two caplets of a supergreen formula, and two whole food multivitamin caplets.

Snacks

raw almonds and apple wedges

whole food nutrition bar with beta-glucans from soluble oat fiber

eight to twelve ounces of water

Before Bed

Exercise: go for a walk outdoors or participate in a favorite sport or recreational activity.

Evening alkalizing drink: mix the following ingredients in twelve ounces of warm purified water: two teaspoons of organic raw apple cider vinegar, one serving of an alkalizing mineral formula with AlkaPlex, and two teaspoons of raw organic honey.

Advanced hygiene: repeat the advanced hygiene instructions from the morning of Day 1.

Emotional health: repeat the emotional health recommendations from Day 1.

Purpose: ask yourself these questions: "Did I live a life of purpose today?" "What did I do to add value to someone else's life today?" Commit to living a day of purpose tomorrow.

Prayer: thank God for this day, asking Him to give you a restoring night's rest and a fresh start tomorrow. Thank Him for His steadfast love that never ceases and His mercies that are new every morning. Read 1 Corinthians 13:4–8 aloud.

Body therapy: spend ten minutes listening to soothing music before you retire.

Sleep: go to bed by 10:30 p.m.

Day 3

Upon Waking

Prayer: thank God because this is the day that the Lord has made. Rejoice and be glad in it. Thank Him for the breath in your lungs and the life in your body. Ask the Lord to heal your body and use your experience to benefit the lives of others. Read Ephesians 6:13–18 aloud.

Purpose: ask the Lord to give you an opportunity to add significance to someone's life today. Watch for that opportunity. Ask God to use you this day for His intended purpose.

Advanced hygiene: follow the advanced hygiene recommendations from the morning of Day 1.

Reduce toxins: follow the recommendations to reduce toxins from the morning of Day 1.

Morning alkalizing drink: mix the following ingredients in twelve ounces of warm purified water: two teaspoons of organic raw apple cider vinegar, one serving of an alkalizing mineral formula with AlkaPlex, and two teaspoons of raw organic honey. (For recommended products, visit www.BiblicalHealthInstitute.com and click on the Resource Guide.)

Body therapy: get twenty minutes of direct sunlight sometime during the day, but be careful between the hours of 10:00 a.m. and 2:00 p.m.

Exercise: perform functional fitness exercises for five to fifteen minutes or spend five to fifteen minutes on a mini trampoline. Finish with five to ten minutes of deep-breathing exercises. (One to three rounds of the exercises can be found at www.BiblicalHealthInstitute.com.)

Emotional health: follow the emotional health recommendations from Day 1.

Breakfast

four to eight ounces of organic whole milk yogurt or cottage cheese with fruit (pineapple, peaches or berries), honey, and a dash of vanilla extract

handful of raw almonds

Drink eight ounces of water.

Supplements: take one capsule of a probiotic/enzyme blend with soil-based organisms, two caplets of a supergreen formula, and two whole food multivitamin caplets.

Lunch

Before eating, drink eight ounces of water.

During lunch, drink eight ounces of water.

large green salad with mixed greens, avocado, carrots, cucumbers, celery, tomatoes, red cabbage, red peppers, red onions, and sprouts with three hard-boiled omega-3 eggs. Caution: if eating certain raw veggies causes a flare-up of heartburn symptoms, make sure to chew very well and eliminate cabbage, peppers, and onions from the salad.

salad dressing: mix extra virgin olive oil, apple cider vinegar or lemon juice, minced fresh garlic, naturally brewed soy sauce, Celtic Sea Salt, herbs, and spices; or, mix one tablespoon of extra virgin olive oil with one tablespoon of a healthy store-bought dressing

one piece of fruit in season

Supplements: take one capsule of a probiotic/enzyme blend with soil-based organisms, two caplets of a supergreen formula, and two whole food multivitamin caplets.

Dinner

(Please note: If you're suffering from heartburn or acid reflux, it is best to finish dinner by 7:30 p.m. or at least three hours before your normal bedtime.)

During dinner, drink eight to sixteen ounces of water.

red meat steak (beef, buffalo, lamb, or venison)

steamed broccoli

baked sweet potato with butter

large green salad with mixed greens, avocado, carrots, cucumbers, celery, tomatoes, red cabbage, red peppers, red onions, and sprouts. Caution: if eating certain raw veggies causes a flare-up of heartburn symptoms, make sure to chew very well and eliminate cabbage, peppers, and onions from the salad.

salad dressing: mix extra virgin olive oil, apple cider vinegar or lemon juice, minced fresh garlic, naturally brewed soy sauce, Celtic Sea Salt, herbs, and spices; or, mix one tablespoon of extra virgin olive oil with one tablespoon of a healthy store-bought dressing

Supplements: take one capsule of a probiotic/enzyme blend with soil-based organisms, two caplets of a supergreen formula, and two whole food multivitamin caplets.

Snacks

four ounces of whole milk yogurt with fruit, honey, and a few almonds

whole food nutrition bar with beta-glucans from soluble oat fiber

eight to twelve ounces of water or hot or iced fresh-brewed tea with honey

Before Bed

Exercise: go for a walk outdoors or participate in a favorite sport or recreational activity.

Evening alkalizing drink: mix the following ingredients in twelve ounces of warm purified water: two teaspoons of organic raw apple cider vinegar, one serving of an alkalizing mineral formula with AlkaPlex, and two teaspoons of raw organic honey. (For recommended products, visit www.BiblicalHealthInstitute.com and click on the Resource Guide.)

Body therapy: take a warm bath for fifteen minutes with eight drops of biblical essential oils added.

Advanced hygiene: follow the advanced hygiene instructions from the morning of Day 1.

Emotional health: follow the forgiveness recommendations from the evening of Day 1.

Purpose: ask yourself these questions: "Did I live a life of purpose today?" "What did I do to add value to someone else's life today?" Commit to living a day of purpose tomorrow.

Prayer: thank God for this day, asking Him to give you a restoring night's rest and a fresh start tomorrow. Thank Him for His steadfast love that never ceases and His mercies that are new every morning. Read Philippians 4:4–8, 11–13, 19 aloud.

Sleep: go to bed by 10:30 p.m.

DAY 4

Upon Waking

Prayer: thank God because this is the day that the Lord has made. Rejoice and be glad in it. Thank Him for the breath in your lungs and the life in your body. Read Matthew 6:9–13 aloud.

Purpose: ask the Lord to give you an opportunity to add significance to someone's life today. Watch for that opportunity. Ask God to use you this day for His intended purpose.

Advanced hygiene: follow the advanced hygiene recommendations from Day 1.

Reduce toxins: follow the recommendations for reducing toxins from Day 1.

Morning alkalizing drink: mix the following ingredients in twelve ounces of warm purified water: two teaspoons of organic raw apple cider vinegar, one serving of an alkalizing mineral formula with AlkaPlex, and two teaspoons of raw organic honey.

Exercise: perform functional fitness exercises for five to fifteen minutes or spend five to fifteen minutes on a mini trampoline. Finish with five to ten minutes of deep-breathing exercises. (One to three rounds of the exercises can be found at www.BiblicalHealthInstitute.com.)

Body therapy: take a hot and cold shower. After a normal shower, alternate sixty seconds of water as hot as you can stand it, followed by sixty seconds of water as cold as you can stand it. Repeat cycle four times for a total of eight minutes, finishing with cold.

Emotional health: follow the emotional health recommendations from the morning of Day 1.

Breakfast

three soft-boiled or poached omega-3 eggs

four ounces of sprouted whole grain cereal with two ounces of whole milk yogurt (for recommended products, visit www.Biblical HealthInstitute.com and click on the Resource Guide)

Drink eight ounces of water.

Supplements: take one capsule of a probiotic/enzyme blend with soil-based organisms, two caplets of a supergreen formula, and two whole food multivitamin caplets.

Lunch

Before eating, drink eight ounces of water.

During lunch, drink eight ounces of water.

large green salad with mixed greens, avocado, carrots, cucumbers, celery, tomatoes, red cabbage, red peppers, red onions, and sprouts with three ounces of low mercury, high omega-3 canned tuna. Caution: if eating certain raw veggies causes a flare-up of heartburn symptoms, make sure to chew very well and eliminate cabbage, peppers, and onions from the salad.

salad dressing: mix extra virgin olive oil, apple cider vinegar or lemon juice, minced fresh garlic, naturally brewed soy sauce, Celtic Sea Salt, herbs, and spices; or, mix one tablespoon of extra virgin olive oil with one tablespoon of a healthy store-bought dressing

one bunch of grapes with seeds

Supplements: take one capsule of a probiotic/enzyme blend with soil-based organisms, two caplets of a supergreen formula, and two whole food multivitamin caplets.

Dinner

(Please note: If you're suffering from heartburn or acid reflux, it is best to finish dinner by 7:30 p.m. or at least three hours before your normal bedtime.)

Drink eight to sixteen ounces of water.

grilled chicken breast

steamed veggies

small portion of cooked nongluten whole grain (quinoa, amaranth, millet, or buckwheat) cooked with one tablespoon of extra virgin coconut oil

large green salad with mixed greens, avocado, carrots, cucumbers, celery, tomatoes, red cabbage, red peppers, red onions, and sprouts. Caution: if eating certain raw veggies causes a flare-up of heartburn symptoms, make sure to chew very well and eliminate cabbage, peppers, and onions from the salad.

salad dressing: mix extra virgin olive oil, apple cider vinegar or lemon juice, minced fresh garlic, naturally brewed soy sauce, Celtic Sea Salt, herbs, and spices; or, mix one tablespoon of extra virgin olive oil with one tablespoon of a healthy store-bought dressing

Supplements: take one capsule of a probiotic/enzyme blend with soil-based organisms, two caplets of a supergreen formula, and two whole food multivitamin caplets.

Snacks

apple and carrots with raw almond butter

whole food nutrition bar with beta-glucans from soluble oat fiber

eight to twelve ounces of water

Before Bed

Drink eight to twelve ounces of water.

Exercise: go for a walk outdoors or participate in a favorite sport or recreational activity.

Evening alkalizing drink: mix the following ingredients in twelve ounces of warm purified water: two teaspoons of organic raw apple cider vinegar, one serving of an alkalizing mineral formula with AlkaPlex, and two teaspoons of raw organic honey.

Advanced hygiene: follow the advanced hygiene recommendations from the morning of Day 1.

Emotional health: follow the forgiveness recommendations from the evening of Day 1.

Purpose: ask yourself these questions: "Did I live a life of purpose today?" "What did I do to add value to someone else's life today?" Commit to living a day of purpose tomorrow.

Prayer: thank God for this day, asking Him to give you a restoring night's rest and a fresh start tomorrow. Thank Him for His steadfast love that never ceases and His mercies that are new every morning. Read Romans 8:35, 37–39 aloud.

Body therapy: spend ten minutes listening to soothing music before you retire.

Sleep: go to bed by 10:30 p.m.

DAY 5 (PARTIAL FAST DAY)

Upon Waking

Prayer: thank God because this is the day that the Lord has made.

Rejoice and be glad in it. Thank Him for the breath in your lungs and the life in your body. Read Isaiah 58:6–9 aloud.

Purpose: ask the Lord to give you an opportunity to add significance to someone's life today. Watch for that opportunity. Ask God to use you this day for His intended purpose.

Advanced hygiene: follow the advanced hygiene recommendations from Day 1.

Reduce toxins: follow the recommendations for reducing toxins from Day 1.

Morning alkalizing drink: mix the following ingredients in twelve ounces of warm purified water: two teaspoons of organic raw apple cider vinegar, one serving of an alkalizing mineral formula with AlkaPlex, and two teaspoons of raw organic honey.

Exercise: perform functional fitness exercises for five to fifteen minutes or spend five to fifteen minutes on a mini trampoline. Finish with five to ten minutes of deep-breathing exercises.

Body therapy: get twenty minutes of direct sunlight sometime during the day, but be careful between the hours of 10:00 a.m. and 2:00 p.m.

Emotional health: follow the emotional health recommendations from the morning of Day 1.

Breakfast

none (partial fast day)

Drink eight to twelve ounces of water.

Supplements: none (partial fast day).

Lunch

none (partial fast day)

Drink eight to twelve ounces of water.

Supplements: none (partial fast day).

Dinner

(Please note: If you're suffering from heartburn or acid reflux, it is best to finish dinner by 7:30 p.m. or at least three hours before your normal bedtime.)

eight to sixteen ounces of water

Heartburn-Bustin' Chicken Soup (see page 17 for the recipe)

cultured vegetables (for recommended products, visit www.Biblical HealthInstitute.com and click on the Resource Guide)

large green salad with mixed greens, avocado, carrots, cucumbers, celery, tomatoes, red cabbage, red peppers, red onions, and sprouts (caution: if eating certain raw veggies causes a flare-up of heartburn symptoms, make sure to chew very well and eliminate cabbage, peppers, and onions from the salad)

salad dressing: mix extra virgin olive oil, apple cider vinegar or lemon juice, minced fresh garlic, naturally brewed soy sauce, Celtic Sea Salt, herbs, and spices; or, mix one tablespoon of extra virgin olive oil with one tablespoon of a healthy store-bought dressing

Supplements: take one capsule of a probiotic/enzyme blend with soil-based organisms, two caplets of a supergreen formula, and two whole food multivitamin caplets.

Snacks

none (partial fast day)

eight ounces of water

Before Bed

Drink eight to twelve ounces of water.

Exercise: go for a walk outdoors or participate in a favorite sport or recreational activity.

Evening alkalizing drink: mix the following ingredients in twelve ounces of warm purified water: two teaspoons of organic raw apple cider vinegar, one serving of an alkalizing mineral formula with AlkaPlex, and two teaspoons of raw organic honey. (For recommended products, visit www.BiblicalHealthInstitute.com and click on the Resource Guide.)

Advanced hygiene: follow the advanced hygiene recommendations from the morning of Day 1.

Emotional health: follow the forgiveness recommendations from the evening of Day 1.

Body therapy: take a warm bath for fifteen minutes with eight drops of biblical essential oils added.

Purpose: ask yourself these questions: "Did I live a life of purpose today?" "What did I do to add value to someone else's life today?" Commit to living a day of purpose tomorrow.

Prayer: thank God for this day, asking Him to give you a restoring night's rest and a fresh start tomorrow. Thank Him for His steadfast love that never ceases and His mercies that are new every morning. Read Isaiah 58:6–9 aloud.

Sleep: go to bed by 10:30 p.m.

DAY 6 (REST DAY)

Upon Waking

Prayer: thank God because this is the day that the Lord has made. Rejoice and be glad in it. Thank Him for the breath in your lungs and the life in your body. Read Psalm 23 aloud.

Purpose: ask the Lord to give you an opportunity to add significance to someone's life today. Watch for that opportunity. Ask God to use you this day for His intended purpose.

Advanced hygiene: follow the advanced hygiene recommendations from Day 1.

Reduce toxins: follow the recommendations for reducing toxins from Day 1.

Morning alkalizing drink: mix the following ingredients in twelve ounces of warm purified water: two teaspoons of organic raw apple cider vinegar, one serving of an alkalizing mineral formula with AlkaPlex, and two teaspoons of raw organic honey. (For recommended products, visit www.BiblicalHealthInstitute.com and click on the Resource Guide.)

Exercise: no formal exercise since it's a rest day.

Body therapies: none since it's a rest day.

Emotional health: follow the emotional health recommendations from the morning of Day 1.

Breakfast

two or three eggs cooked any style in one tablespoon of extra virgin coconut oil

one grapefruit or orange

handful of almonds

Drink eight ounces of water.

Supplements: take one capsule of a probiotic/enzyme blend with soil-based organisms, two caplets of a supergreen formula, and two whole food multivitamin caplets.

Lunch

Drink eight to sixteen ounces of water.

large green salad with mixed greens, avocado, carrots, cucumbers, celery, tomatoes, red cabbage, red peppers, red onions, and sprouts with two ounces of low mercury, high omega-3 canned tuna (caution: if eating certain raw veggies causes a flare-up of heartburn symptoms, make sure to chew very well and eliminate cabbage, peppers, and onions from the salad)

salad dressing: mix extra virgin olive oil, apple cider vinegar or lemon juice, minced fresh garlic, naturally brewed soy sauce, Celtic Sea Salt, herbs, and spices; or, mix one tablespoon of extra virgin olive oil with one tablespoon of a healthy store-bought dressing

one organic apple with the skin

Supplements: take one capsule of a probiotic/enzyme blend with soil-based organisms, two caplets of a supergreen formula, and two whole food multivitamin caplets.

Dinner

(Please note: If you're suffering from heartburn or acid reflux, it is best to finish dinner by 7:30 p.m. or at least three hours before your normal bedtime.)

Drink eight to sixteen ounces of water.

roasted organic chicken

cooked vegetables (carrots, onions, peas, etc.)

large green salad with mixed greens, avocado, carrots, cucumbers, celery, tomatoes, red cabbage, red peppers, red onions, and sprouts (caution: if eating certain raw veggies causes a flare-up of heartburn symptoms, make sure to chew very well and eliminate cabbage, peppers, and onions from the salad)

salad dressing: mix extra virgin olive oil, apple cider vinegar or lemon juice, minced fresh garlic, naturally brewed soy sauce, Celtic Sea Salt, herbs, and spices; or, mix one tablespoon of extra virgin olive oil with one tablespoon of a healthy store-bought dressing

Supplements: take one capsule of a probiotic/enzyme blend with soil-based organisms, two caplets of a supergreen formula, and two whole food multivitamin caplets.

Snacks

handful of raw almonds with apple wedges

whole food nutrition bar with beta-glucans from soluble oat fiber

eight to twelve ounces of water or hot or iced fresh-brewed tea with honey

Before Bed

Drink eight to twelve ounces of water.

Exercise: go for a walk outdoors or participate in a favorite sport or recreational activity.

Evening alkalizing drink: mix the following ingredients in twelve ounces of warm purified water: two teaspoons of organic raw apple cider vinegar, one serving of an alkalizing mineral formula with AlkaPlex, and two teaspoons of raw organic honey.

Advanced hygiene: follow the advanced hygiene recommendations from the morning of Day 1.

Emotional health: follow the forgiveness recommendations from the evening of Day 1.

Purpose: ask yourself these questions: "Did I live a life of purpose today?" "What did I do to add value to someone else's life today?" Commit to living a day of purpose tomorrow.

Prayer: thank God for this day, asking Him to give you a restoring night's rest and a fresh start tomorrow. Thank Him for His steadfast love that never ceases and His mercies that are new every morning. Read Psalm 23 aloud.

Body therapy: spend ten minutes listening to soothing music before you retire.

Sleep: go to bed by 10:30 p.m.

DAY 7

Upon Waking

Prayer: thank God because this is the day that the Lord has made. Rejoice and be glad in it. Thank Him for the breath in your lungs and the life in your body. Read Psalm 91 aloud.

Purpose: ask the Lord to give you an opportunity to add significance to someone's life today. Watch for that opportunity. Ask God to use you this day for His intended purpose.

Advanced hygiene: follow the advanced hygiene recommendations from Day 1.

Reduce toxins: follow the recommendations for reducing toxins from Day 1.

Morning alkalizing drink: mix the following ingredients in twelve ounces of warm purified water: two teaspoons of organic raw apple cider vinegar, one serving of an alkalizing mineral formula with AlkaPlex, and two teaspoons of raw organic honey.

Exercise: perform functional fitness exercises for five to fifteen minutes or spend five to fifteen minutes on a mini trampoline. Finish with five to ten minutes of deep-breathing exercises.

Body therapy: get twenty minutes of direct sunlight sometime during the day, but be careful between the hours of 10:00 a.m. and 2:00 p.m.

Emotional health: follow the emotional health recommendations from the morning of Day 1.

Breakfast

Make a smoothie in a blender with the following ingredients:

1 cup plain yogurt or kefir (goat's milk is best)

1 tablespoon organic flaxseed oil

1 tablespoon organic raw honey

1 cup organic fruit (berries, banana, peaches, pineapple, etc.)

2 tablespoons goat's milk protein powder

dash of vanilla extract (optional)

Supplements: take one capsule of a probiotic/enzyme blend with soil-based organisms, two caplets of a supergreen formula, and two whole food multivitamin caplets.

Lunch

Drink eight to sixteen ounces of water.

large green salad with mixed greens, avocado, carrots, cucumbers, celery, tomatoes, red cabbage, red peppers, red onions, and sprouts with three ounces of cold, poached, or canned wild-caught salmon (caution: if eating certain raw veggies causes a flare-up of heartburn symptoms, make sure to chew very well and eliminate cabbage, peppers, and onions from the salad)

salad dressing: mix extra virgin olive oil, apple cider vinegar or lemon juice, minced fresh garlic, naturally brewed soy sauce, Celtic Sea Salt, herbs, and spices; or, mix one tablespoon of extra virgin olive oil with one tablespoon of a healthy store-bought dressing.

one piece of fruit in season

Supplements: take one capsule of a probiotic/enzyme blend with soil-based organisms, two caplets of a supergreen formula, and two whole food multivitamin caplets.

Dinner

(Please note: If you're suffering from heartburn or acid reflux, it is best to finish dinner by 7:30 p.m. or at least three hours before your normal bedtime.)

Drink eight to sixteen ounces of water.

baked or grilled fish of your choice

steamed broccoli

baked sweet potato with butter

large green salad with mixed greens, avocado, carrots, cucumbers, celery, tomatoes, red cabbage, red peppers, red onions, and sprouts (caution: if eating certain raw veggies causes a flare-up of heartburn symptoms, make sure to chew very well and eliminate cabbage, peppers, and onions from the salad)

salad dressing: mix extra virgin olive oil, apple cider vinegar or lemon juice, minced fresh garlic, naturally brewed soy sauce, Celtic Sea

Salt, herbs, and spices; or, mix one tablespoon of extra virgin olive oil with one tablespoon of a healthy store-bought dressing

Supplements: take one capsule of a probiotic/enzyme blend with soil-based organisms, two caplets of a supergreen formula, and two whole food multivitamin caplets.

Snacks

apple slices with raw sesame butter (tahini)

whole food nutrition bar with beta-glucans from soluble oat fiber

eight to twelve ounces of water

Before Bed

Drink eight to twelve ounces of water or hot tea with honey.

Exercise: go for a walk outdoors or participate in a favorite sport or recreational activity.

Evening alkalizing drink: mix the following ingredients in twelve ounces of warm purified water: two teaspoons of organic raw apple cider vinegar, one serving of an alkalizing mineral formula with AlkaPlex, and two teaspoons of raw organic honey. (For recommended products, visit www.BiblicalHealthInstitute.com and click on the Resource Guide.)

Advanced hygiene: follow the advanced hygiene recommendations from the morning of Day 1.

Emotional health: follow the forgiveness recommendations from the evening of Day 1.

Body therapy: take a warm bath for fifteen minutes with eight drops of biblical essential oils added.

Purpose: ask yourself these questions: "Did I live a life of purpose today?" "What did I do to add value to someone else's life today?" Commit to living a day of purpose tomorrow.

Prayer: thank God for this day, asking Him to give you a restoring night's rest and a fresh start tomorrow. Thank Him for His steadfast love that never ceases and His mercies that are new every morning. Read 1 Corinthians 13:4–8 aloud.

Sleep: go to bed by 10:30 p.m.

Day 8 and Beyond

If you're feeling better, you can repeat the Great Physician's Rx for Heartburn and Acid Reflux Battle Plan as many times as you'd like. For detailed step-by-step suggestions and meal and lifestyle plans, visit www.GreatPhysiciansRx.com and join the 40 Day Health Experience for continued good health. Or you may be interested in the Lifetime of Wellness plan if you want to maintain your newfound level of health. These online programs will provide you with customized daily meal and exercise plans and give you the tools to track your progress.

If you've experienced positive results from the Great Physician's prescription for heartburn and acid reflux program, I encourage you to reach out to people you know and recommend this book and program to them. You can learn how to lead a small group at your church or home by visiting www.BiblicalHealthInstitute.com.

Remember, you don't have to be a doctor or a health expert to help transform the life of someone you care about—you just have to be willing.

Allow me to offer this prayer of blessing paraphrased from Numbers 6:24–26 to you:

May the Lord bless you and keep you
May the Lord make His face to shine upon you and be gracious unto you
May the Lord lift up His countenance upon you and bring you peace
In the name of Yeshua Ha Mashiach, Jesus our Messiah

Amen

Need Recipes?

For a detailed list of over two hundred healthy and delicious recipes contained in the Great Physician's Rx eating plan, please visit www.BiblicalHealthInstitute.com.

NOTES

Introduction

1. Sharon Gillson, "Heartburn Fast Facts," About.com, http://heartburn.about.com/od/understandingheartburn/a/hrtbrnfastfacts.htm (accessed April 5, 2007).

2. "Advice from the Experts," National Heartburn Alliance, http://www.heartburnalliance.org/section2/index_textonly.jsp (accessed April 5, 2007).

3. "Quotations: Ayurvedic Concepts," Quote Garden, http://www.quotegarden.com/ayurveda.html (accessed April 5, 2007).

4. Steve Jackson, "Super Bowl Deserves to Become National Holiday," *Michigan Daily,* January 27, 2003.

5. D. Lindsey Berkson, *Healthy Digestion the Natural Way* (New York: John Wiley & Sons, 2000), 59.

6. Penni Crabtree, "Me-Too Medicines," *San Diego Union-Tribune,* November 20, 2005.

7. "Prilosec OTC, Actress Marg Helgenburger and Thousands of Women Roll the Dice to Raise Money for Breast Cancer Research," *PR Newswire,* February 10, 2006, http://phx.corporate-ir.net/phoenix.zhtml?c=104574&p=irol-newsArticle_Print&ID=815622&highlight= (accessed on April 11, 2007).

8. Gardiner Harris, "2 New Fronts in Heartburn Market Battle," *New York Times,* August 20, 2003.

9. Reuters News Service, "Acupoint Stimulation Promising for Heartburn," September 12, 2005.

10. *Encyclopedia of Natural Healing* (Burnaby, B.C., Canada: Alive Publishing Group, 1997), 807–8.

Key #1

1. Rex Russell, *What the Bible Says About Healthy Living* (Ventura, CA: Regal, 1996), 62–63.

2. "High-Fiber Diet May Halt Heartburn: Fiber Protects Against GERD, Study Shows," WebMD.com, http://www.webmd.com/heartburn-gerd/news/20050105/high-fiber-diet-may-halt-heartburn, (accessed April 11, 2007).

3. Tom Cowan, M.D., "Ask the Doctor About Gastroesophageal Reflux Disease (GERD)," Ask the Doctor, http://www.westonaprice.org/askdoctor/gerd.html (accessed April 11, 2007).

4. Kathleen Donnelly, "The Long and Tortured History of Heartburn," MSN, http://health.msn.com/centers/heartburnandgerd/articlepage.aspx?cp-documentid=100125483 (accessed April 5, 2007).

5. Kaayla T. Daniel, MS, CCN, "Why Broth Is Beautiful—'Essential' Roles for Proline, Glycine and Gelatin," The Weston A. Price Foundation, http://www.westonaprice.org/foodfeatures/brothisbeautiful.html (accessed April 5, 2007).

6. F. M. Pottenger, "Hydrophilic Colloid Diet," *Health and Healing Wisdom*, 21 (Spring 1997): 1, 17.

7. F. Batmanghelidj, M.D., *You're Not Sick, You're Thirsty!* (New York: Warner Books, 2003), 131.

8. Ibid., 132.

9. D. W. Murphy and D. O. Castell, "Chocolate and Heartburn: Evidence of Increased Esophageal Acid Exposure After Chocolate Ingestion," *American Journal of Gastroenterology* 83, no. 6 (June 1988): 633–36.

10. R. Fass, American College of Chest Physicians, "Predictors of Heartburn During Sleep in a Large Prospective Cohort Study," *Chest* 127 (May 2005): 1658–66.

Key #2

1. Natasha Trenev, "Longevity and the Importance of *L. Bulgaricus* Supplementation," Natren, http://www.natren.com/pages/natashart2.asp (accessed April 5, 2007).

2. Larry Trivieri Jr., ed., *Alternative Medicine: The Definitive Guide* (Berkeley, Calif.: Celestial Arts, 2002), 717.

Key #4

1. PR NewsWire, "New Exercise and Exertion-Related Heartburn Condition Gives New Meaning to 'Feeling the Burn' This Spring," March 23, 2005, Medical News Service, http://medicalnewsservice.com/fullstory.cfm?storyID=2951&fback=yes (accessed April 5, 2007).

2. R. Morgan Griffin, "Tips for Sleep Without Heartburn," WebMD, http://www.webmd.com/content/Article/112/110345.htm?printing=true (accessed April 5, 2007).

Key #5

1. "Misdiagnosis of Medication Causes of Heartburn," Wrong Diagnosis?, http://www.wrongdiagnosis.com/h/heartburn/medic.htm (accessed April 5, 2007).

2. Elaine Gottschall, *Breaking the Vicious Cycle* (Baltimore and Ontario: Kirkton Press, 2004), 24.

3. "Body Burden: The Pollution in People," Environmental Working Group, http://www.ewg.org/sites/humantoxome/ (accessed April 11, 2007).

4. David Steinman and Samuel S. Epstein, M.D., *The Safe Shopper's Bible* (New York: Wiley Publishing, 1995), 18.

ABOUT THE AUTHORS

Jordan Rubin has dedicated his life to transforming the health of God's people one life at a time. He is the founder and chairman of Garden of Life, Inc., a health and wellness company based in West Palm Beach, Florida, that produces organic functional foods, whole food nutritional supplements and personal care products, and he is a much-in-demand speaker on various health topics.

He and his wife, Nicki, are the parents of a toddler-aged son, Joshua. They make their home in Palm Beach Gardens, Florida.

Joseph D. Brasco, M.D., who has extensive knowledge and experience in gastroenterology and internal medicine, attended medical school at Medical College of Wisconsin in Milwaukee, Wisconsin, and is board certified with the American Board of Internal Medicine. Besides writing for various medical journals, he is also the coauthor of *Restoring Your Digestive Health* with Jordan Rubin. Dr. Brasco is currently in private practice in Huntsville, Alabama.

BHI

BIBLICAL HEALTH
INSTITUTE

The Biblical Health Institute (www.BiblicalHealthInstitute.com) is an online learning community housing educational resources and curricula reinforcing and expanding on Jordan Rubin's Biblical Health message.

Biblical Health Institute provides:

1. "101" level **FREE**, introductory courses corresponding to Jordan's book The Great Physician's Rx for Health and Wellness and its seven keys; Current "101" courses include:

   * "Eating to Live 101"

   * "Whole Food Nutrition Supplements 101"

   * "Advanced Hygiene 101"

   * "Exercise and Body Therapies 101"

   * "Reducing Toxins 101"

   * "Emotional Health 101"

   * "Prayer and Purpose 101"

2. **FREE** resources (healthy recipes, what to E.A.T., resource guide)

3. **FREE** media--videos and video clips of Jordan, music therapy samples, etc.--and much more!

Additionally, Biblical Health Institute also offers in-depth courses for those who want to go deeper.

Course offerings include:

   * 40-hour certificate program to become a Biblical Health Coach

   * A la carte course offerings designed for personal study and growth

   * Home school courses developed by Christian educators, supporting home-schooled students and their parents (designed for middle school and high school ages)

For more information and updates on these and other resources go to
www.BiblicalHealthInstitute.com

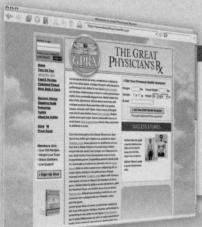